'In addressing human sexuality and its manifold expressions, this book demonstrates that talking about a person's sexual needs can be a profoundly caring act and a deeply humanising process. In exploring the sexual self with compassion, respect and openness, Danuta's reflections on the subject help us to understand more about who we are and what matters to us. After reading this book it is very hard to imagine how anyone could offer person-centred dementia care without considering the sexual needs and sexual identities of people living with a dementia.'

— *Luke Tanner, body psychotherapist*
and dementia care trainer

'Sexuality in older adults, and more specifically people living with dementia, is often not discussed openly. It is a topic that can hold stigma and prejudice. Danuta must be applauded for her sensitive and insightful book – it is refreshing and will go a long way to lifting the lid on a subject that is often dismissed and taboo. Well done and thank you Danuta! A must-read for everyone.'

— *Karen Borochowitz,*
DementiaSA (www.dementisa.org) and
Stuward (www.stuward.com)

Dementia, Sex and Wellbeing

A Person-Centred Guide for People with Dementia, Their Partners, Caregivers and Professionals

Danuta Lipinska

Foreword by Caroline Baker
Afterword by Sally Knocker

Jessica Kingsley *Publishers*
London and Philadelphia

First published in 2018
by Jessica Kingsley Publishers
73 Collier Street
London N1 9BE, UK
and
400 Market Street, Suite 400
Philadelphia, PA 19106, USA

www.jkp.com

Library of Congress Cataloging in Publication Data
A CIP catalog record for this book is available from the Library of Congress

British Library Cataloguing in Publication Data
A CIP catalogue record for this book is available from the British Library

ISBN 978 1 78592 157 5
eISBN 978 1 78450 425 0

Printed and bound in Great Britain

To lovers everywhere

Contents

Foreword

There have been many papers and articles published in recent years about sexuality in dementia care, but have they made us any wiser? Or perhaps more importantly, have they managed to change any of our attitudes or approaches to sexuality and wellbeing in dementia care?

I will begin the foreword for this wonderful book by making a confession. I have worked in dementia care for over thirty years, but began my career as a very young care assistant working on a dementia care ward at a psychiatric hospital. One morning, I was assisting a trained member of staff in changing the sheets on a gentleman's bed, and we were rolling him towards us so that the sheet underneath him could be removed. As we were doing this, I remember being completely horrified at the erection that not only presented itself towards me but pressed against my thigh as I was supporting him.

I remember feeling so embarrassed that I obviously flushed, and I recall that the nurse I was helping not only laughed at me but laughed and joked with the gentleman in the bed that she was glad that he had 'still got it in him', at which point he joined me in looking embarrassed. I was at a complete loss as to what to say or do.

How I wish that this book had been written back then so that I could have gone home and read it! In fact, if I had read it before I had started, then I feel sure that the experience would not have been an issue and I would have approached it (and understood it) quite differently. Many years later, having been qualified for a number of years, I attended a Dementia Care Mapping™ course in Bradford, led by the late Tom Kitwood. The course was enlightening in many ways and I remembered with horror how I had completely ignored that gentleman and virtually ran from the room when his care was complete.

I mention this for two reasons. First, because I had used more malignant social psychology than you could shake a stick at. It wasn't that I said anything or did anything, but that I didn't say or do anything to reassure the gentleman who was obviously very embarrassed. Second, Kitwood raised new thoughts for me about sexuality and dementia care and the need for people to feel close to others – not necessarily the need for sexual contact, but that for comfort and love.

The book you are about to read provides a wealth of information about the sexual needs of us all, not just those living with dementia. It also helps us to question our own values and beliefs about how we might respond in different situations. As I explored each chapter, I couldn't help but try and respond to the reflective questions at the end. As I did, I realised that some of my thoughts had changed and that, after each chapter, I had learned something new that would help me approach my role a little bit differently.

As a dementia professional, you are often asked to provide 'advice' for situations relating to 'incidents' where sexual acts, or people appearing to be 'overly friendly', are being acted out or thought about. For the most part, I think back to Kitwood's ideas and explain the need for comfort and attachment, as well as the 'seven domains of wellbeing' which include the need for connectedness, meaning, growth and joy (Power 2014). Many times though, I simply do not have an answer and we continue to consult with the person (if we are able) and with relatives, carry out capacity and risk assessments, write care plans and try to 'protect the vulnerable'. Even this process can be difficult at times, as any discussions around sex or intimacy are still taboo for some in society.

I would never consider myself an expert in this area. Though she claims not to be, the author of this book clearly is, and she gives us differing ways of exploring this important topic. The case studies that are provided are really helpful in helping us to understand all aspects of dementia, sex and wellbeing, and the points for reflection could also be used as part of an informative discussion or training session with staff. Having read the book, I would like to rename it *Dementia, Sex and Wellbeing: Food for Thought!*

Caroline Baker
Director of Dementia Care at Barchester Healthcare

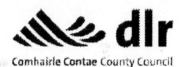

Comhairle Contae County Council

Dun Laoghaire Rathdown Libraries
Dear Borrower

Items that you have returned

Title: The pearl thief / Fiona McIntosh.
ID: DLR5000032929

Title: The survivors / Jane Harper.
ID: DLR26000018708

Total items: 2
07/02/2022 12:18

Thank you for using the SelfCheck System.
GD02

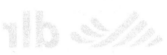

Acknowledgements

There are so many people and experiences over the years that have influenced the writing of this book and I am so grateful for the life and abundant blessings that have brought me this far.

In particular, I offer enormous thanks to the women and men living with dementia, their partners and families who have shared with me and at such depth, with grace, humour, joy and sorrow, as clients in counselling, in support groups, care homes and day centres over two continents and over 30 years. I hope that I have learned well from all you had to teach me, and that together we can pass on the baton.

Thanks to the hundreds of professionals who attended training sessions and shared their stories and their willingness to engage with Self and enhance their practice with regard to people living with dementia and sex. You are all part of this book.

Thank you, dear John Killick, for those early conversations, encouragement and the invitation to write 'Sexually Speaking' in *Pathways* newsletter for the Dementia Services Development Centre at Stirling University – the beginning of putting it all on paper.

Professor Brian Thorne, my mentor and friend who smiled knowingly when I vowed never to write again and offered warmth, wisdom and encouragement over many olives.

I am so appreciative of the time, kindness and generosity of those who have read the book and have encouraged others to do the same.

Carole Evans, who took a chance on my ability to offer training in 1996 and who meticulously read and re-read this manuscript. Thank you – your comments were invaluable and your friendship is a treasured gift.

Dr Caroline Baker, for sharing her considerable expertise, generous appraisal and encouragement, and Sally Knocker, for her honest reflections, humour and warmth. There can be no better way to begin and end a book!

Mary Purnell, my seaside supervisor – thank you for helping me to keep the 'big picture' in view and the person-centred approach alive and well.

My 'Noddfa' family in North Wales loved and cared for me and cheered me on through the earliest chapters with joy and enthusiasm and the gifts of place, presence and prayer.

A huge thank you to Jessica Kingsley Publishers, without whom this would not have happened. In particular, my gratitude to Dr Natalie Watson, who captured the vision and the possibility of this book and held me and it together over the months, and to Daisy Watts and Victoria Peters for all the detail.

Thank you is too brief an acknowledgement for the unswerving belief and support of my husband John and my loving family and friends, who knew this book, too, was destined for the world.

With gratitude, humility and love,
Danuta Lipinska,
Norwich 2017

Introduction

This book has been a long time coming. It has been a constant companion throughout all of my nursing, counselling, and training relationships since my early days as a student nurse beginning in 1974.

Our human relationships and sexual selves can encompass great emotions and many memories, not all of them positive. Yet throughout my long and interesting professional life it seems to me that this is an area that receives little positive attention and not much, until recently, in the form of professional training across the counselling, health and social care professions. I knew that there was still something to be shared on this topic and I trust that I will have at least created an overview and an introduction.

Meeting more women and men living with dementia, many of whom are under the age of 60, I have felt a particular urgency to write about these experiences and create space for conversations as part of our attempts to support people to live well with dementia.

Of course, it is also a part of my life and my future. It may well be part of yours and the person you support. It is my hope that my shared experiences will resonate with you, will encourage reminiscence, and will stimulate new ideas and possibilities.

Let me say from the outset that this book is not the answer to everyone's questions about dementia, sex and wellbeing. It is merely an attempt to share the questions I have been asked or have asked myself in my long career. It is an opportunity to share some of the explorations and conversations, and for you to do the same as you read. It may be that we both stir up yet another batch of questions – as I have already discovered as I began writing. Despite the wealth of publications across all aspects of living with dementia, diagnosis and care, very little exists that addresses sex, dementia and wellbeing in the same sentence.

The title of this book is designed to encourage us to think differently about sex and dementia and offer the possibility that, in fact, the experience of wellbeing in conjunction with these other words need not be thought of as unusual or strange bedfellows.

You could be asking the question, 'Well, why would it be strange to imagine that people living with dementia may still want to engage in sex?' You could also be saying, 'I have never really thought about this', or 'This is not part of my life now.' If you are posing these questions and anything else in between, then I hope you might find something of interest in these few pages.

The definition of 'strange bedfellows', according to the Oxford Dictionary, is 'unlikely companions/allies, odd, unlikely'. This notion, for many, may be how they perceive or imagine this area of human relating, functioning and expressing when placed side by side with the word 'dementia'. The right to freedom of expression, including sexuality, is a basic human right and requires inclusion in the lives of all men and women for whom neurology, age, race, culture, sexual preference, gender, socio-economic status, spirituality or disability might dictate otherwise.

Supporting women and men living with dementia requires greater openness and willingness to consider how much more we share than we differ. We are fortunate at this point in our discussions that people living with dementia are taking centre stage in their own lives and letting us know what is and is not helpful and important to them. Lucy Whitman's book *People with Dementia Speak Out* (2016) is one vivid example. When I spoke to men and women living with dementia about this book, they have been unanimously interested and adamant that the book must be written and that these conversations and deliberations are important and necessary and have long been neglected.

The experiences of sexuality, sex and intimacy are as important for the person with dementia as is the need for person-centred care, sensitive communication and validation. It is part of our identity, after all. My intention is to view adult sexuality and the need for intimacy and belonging as affected by living with dementia.

My first book, *Person-Centred Counselling for People with Dementia: Making Sense of Self* (2009), presented the experiences I gathered as a counsellor both in the USA and UK. It describes the therapeutic relationship and the importance of being able to offer counselling to men and women living with dementia if they would like it.

This book is being written seven years on and is partly a response to many questions raised by people living with dementia, their partners and the professionals who support them.

It is also important to note that for many people the sexual can only be expressed in a loving relationship. We pursue love and are pursued by love regardless of age, gender, sexual preference, socio-economic status, political persuasion, race, abilities, distance and even death. Our love of love and the need for romantic love and intimacy in our lives reach beyond the physical and the sexual and can take many forms. I have separated love from sex here, because it is too easy to link love and sex and create a romantic scenario where one may not exist, and that may not be everyone's preferred experience. It is essential to remember, too, that, for some people, love and sex may be part of an intricate abusive situation, past and/or present.

The assumptions we may make based on our own unique perspective – about love, sex, intimacy and romance – are not the same for everyone and do not necessarily co-exist. Some may even find it easier when they don't. I would like the reader to be able to use their own definitions for whatever best reflects their lifestyle and their experience. For some of us, the best sex we ever had was not with someone we were in love with. For some of us, the best loving relationships are non-sexual. Others have found love and sex works well for them. For others, the best is yet to come. These are all enticing considerations for another time. In our support of those living with dementia, it is important to remember that love, belonging and intimacy of the non-sexual variety are also part of life and are all valuable experiences. But there is more. As one colleague at a workshop shared, 'Sometimes you just want sex.' If that is the case, we must be truthful, at least to ourselves, about what is being replaced, what is a distraction to the underlying need.

Professionals are often skilled at offering what might look and feel like the sense of non-sexual love, friendship, belonging, sensuality and intimacy to people we support, and long may it continue. However, we need to stay person-centred and willing to focus on what may be the other person's reality. What do we say and do when it comes right down to sex? When I ask care staff in a training session, 'When and under what circumstances can someone else decide that you can no longer have sex?', the answer from hundreds of women and men, over many years and across two continents, is invariably an emphatic 'no one' and 'never'. And yet, without even thinking, we ignore sexuality in the lives of older people and people living with dementia, and thereby make decisions on their behalf, by not including the possibilities in our thinking and feeling. When we do include their sexuality in our thought processes, resulting in holistic and person-centred approaches, we are truly embracing the whole person. We can confidently create opportunities for conversations to develop with persons and their partners if they have them, and with care staff and other professionals.

What do we say and do when there is a great need for the physical connection to Self and/or other(s)? When only the delight and release of orgasm will do; when there is a great longing to be filled and/or to fill another with all that we are and can be in that moment? There is great power and autonomy, control and potency, achievement and self-directed pleasure involved in sex. These states can also define many of the aspects of Self that begin to diminish when living with dementia.

The need for these conversations and this book is in response to my experiences that living with dementia often alters a person's ability to continue to make choices that are a deeply personal and meaningful part of their identity, quality of life and wellbeing. Sexuality, sex, intimacy and sensuality are aspects of identity often taken for granted when we are well-functioning adults. The absence of or changes to these aspects of living may not herald significant loss for many, but for most adults it is likely to cause concern and often feelings of inadequacy, impotence, low self-esteem, grief and depression. But for men and women living with dementia, in partnership or single, who wish to continue to enjoy their sex lives despite neurology or diminished expectations, I believe a new approach is needed. The book is written primarily for professionals, lovers and families. I hope that people living with dementia will also find value here and a true reflection of some of their concerns, feelings and issues. I will attempt to give examples of my experiences by using scenarios and narratives that have emerged from real life and relationships. For me, it also makes sense that together we might find new and positive ways to address sexuality within the context of living well with dementia and to normalise those conversations. This will require a brave, open, person-centred approach which sees wellbeing and self-actualisation as complementary.

For some, there may currently be an unexpressed concern that this wonderful part of life will become invisible, ignored and allowed to wither and rot, or become a 'problem to be managed or dealt with' – and, heaven forbid, by your adult children.

Adult children find it especially challenging and emotionally complex to think about their parent or relative as a sexual being with rights and needs as well as care needs. It may be a cause for even more concern and rock the family boat if a parent has found a new partner while Mum or Dad is living at the nursing home, and discretion may be the better part of valour in this scenario.

Some adult children are happy for their parent if the person themselves seems happy, and no one is being hurt or exploited. In any relationship where affection, sex and love are shared, if it ends with illness, leaving the environment or death, then our continued challenge is to support that person through their loss and grief and provide an alternative focus.

John and Elaine, brother and sister, have brought their mother Jenny, 79, to live at a care home. Their dad died three years ago, and Jenny's vascular dementia seemed to get much worse in a short space of time. Our conversation went something along these lines.

'We talked earlier about the many changes that happen with dementia and how those affect living with others – initially, strangers in a strange place. Some of those changes occur in how the brain deals with sexual feelings, thoughts and behaviour, or just the very human need to feel close and affectionate with someone. We know that for some people it may be difficult to keep those needs under wraps at times, since the brain may not remember that they are usually private or with people we know. We try our best to notice when someone might become more upset, sad and withdrawn or frustrated or even aggressive, or says and does things of a sexual nature. We will try to maintain that person's dignity and privacy as best we can, and offer other things to distract them, take their minds off it and offer activities we know they enjoy to let off a bit of steam. It will never replace a person's sex life, but it might help someone feel more in control and that there are other things that can give them pleasure and feel part of a close and caring connection.'

D: It's not always comfortable talking about sex, especially when it's about your mother, and your mother has dementia. Private things of all sorts might not stay private. You have said that your parents had a good marriage. I imagine that may have included sex.

J: I've never thought about it before. To be honest, you don't like to think of your parents having a sex life. But I suppose they must have, eh, Elaine? At least twice, as far as we know.

E: This is so hard to think about and talk about. But I suppose it's better to imagine now that if things did kick off, we would know how you would support her and that we would know you were taking care of her, keeping her safe and not letting her annoy anybody else either.

J: Does it happen a lot, then?

D: No, not really, but it can and does, and we want to be aware and sensitive to your mother's needs and see how we can best support her.

E: Well, don't phone me up and tell me she's in bed with another resident. I don't want to know. It would break my heart. It's still her life, and I don't need to know about all of it once she is living here. I want her to be happy, whatever that means, if nobody gets hurt.

J: Yeah, I'm fine with that, too.

This situation may never arise for Elaine and John and their mother, but nor will it come as a complete shock or a surprise if it does. Elaine and John will know that the manager and the staff will have been trained to be sensitive and observant and will have learned about their mother's life and will be able to respond appropriately. They will know that they can trust that the staff will be aware of human beings' need for touch and comfort and a sense of connection and affection.

They will be assured that these will be offered in non-sexual and non-threatening ways and that they will respond in caring ways towards Jenny should she let them know or they discover that this is something she needs and enjoys. Should Jenny wish to have a more intimate and sexual relationship with another resident, Elaine and John will know that, as far as possible, everything will be done to ensure their mother's safety, dignity and privacy in the first instance, and that of other residents too.

It would be a mistake, however, to assume that persons with dementia do not share the general population's views about sex in later life and talking about their own sexual experiences. We are still apparently better at talking about other people's sex lives than our own, even to our own sexual partners.

I do not mean to imply that everyone everywhere should have a fabulous sex life or, indeed, even want one at all. There are people for whom sex is not all it's made out to be, for whatever reasons. There are people who would rather go for a long walk with the dog or indulge in a box-set marathon of their favourite TV show with a bowl of popcorn.

This area of interest in the brain and sex and ageing is not new. Its connection with dementia, however, is more recent. I have been impressed for many years by the way in which the learning disabilities community has addressed the important issues of sexual rights, health, safe sex, dating, contraception and the breadth of sexualities. Have a look at the websites of BILD, the British Institute of Learning Disabilities (www.bild.org.uk) and the mental health charity Mind (www.mind.org.uk). It occurs to me that if we are comparing the challenges to cognition and behaviour and potential for recovery, more similarities than differences exist between the two groups based on brain and behaviour. The

Traumatic Brain Injury website (www.traumaticbraininjury. com) also describes the challenges to sexual behaviour and intimacy, citing most of the same issues that affect persons with dementia and proposing practical solutions. Why, then, is there a deficit of similar open and straightforward information and support for persons with dementia on any of the dementia-specific websites?

The major English-speaking websites for Alzheimer's disease have mostly devoted their information on relationships, intimacy and sex to the heterosexual caregiver as partner. They affirm the need and right to intimate and sexual relationships with our partner as a fulfilling aspect of life lived with dementia. However, if I was living with dementia, where would I look to find information, help or support about my own sexuality, whether in a relationship or single, and the changes dementia might cause? The current language assumes that the behaviour of the person with dementia will be mainly negative, aggressive, problematic, inappropriate and demanding towards the prospective partner. There is obviously more we need to do to change the language and context of what is available for those living with a dementia themselves.

Although this is, of course, important, we know that it is not the whole story of our multiple sexualities and relationships. Of course, there is neither time nor space to address each of them on a website, as is the case here too, but how are LGBTQI (lesbian, gay, bisexual, transgender, queer or questioning, and intersex) people addressed? A brief review of the current state of affairs does show several recent publications. I refer you to the excellent 2015 report by University of Worcester Association of Dementia Studies in partnership with DEEP – Dementia Engagement and Empowerment Project – which specifically sets out to hear the voices of LGBTQI people living with dementia or of partners and friends. The Care Quality Commission (2017) has made a recommitment to equality and diversity in their inspection process. Their focus in year 1, 2017–2018, is to assess 'how providers ensure person-centred care for lesbian, gay, bisexual and transgender (LGBT) people who use adult social care and mental health inpatient services, for people with dementia in acute hospitals and older BME [black and minority ethnic] people using GP practices' (2017).

The recent work of the National Care Forum to highlight LGBTQI needs in care is encouraging. *Lesbian, Gay, Bisexual and Trans* Individuals Living with Dementia* (Westwood and Price 2016) covers a range of important issues, is multidisciplinary and includes the views of international academics and people living with dementia who are lesbian, gay, bisexual or trans. Professor Murna Downs from the University of Bradford has pronounced it 'a milestone in our field'.

In the 2000s I was privileged to run a support group for two years for lesbian, gay and bisexual carers of persons living with dementia. This was a particularly enlightening experience for which I will always be grateful. I developed a new and necessary sensitivity to those carers who so often felt invisible, undermined by the socio-medical establishment, whose voices, if not unheard altogether, were yet a faint whisper from behind the scenes. As I write, these voices are no longer quiet, but strong and full, determined to call us out into relationships that march to a different tune – their own.

When I knew that I was ready to write this book, I ran a workshop at a conference and asked participants what they would like to see in a book of this title. Of many helpful suggestions, one very important request was that the book not be written from a purely heteronormative perspective. As a straight woman, this will be a challenge. I am only able to share my own authentic experiences and those may be limited to only a handful of coloured strands. There are numerous colours and textures to this particular tapestry of sex, dementia and wellbeing, and my hope is that by sharing what I have learned, you will bring your own strands and weave them into the bigger work that will be co-created, side by side. Perhaps it will validate your already enlightened views and professional practice and encourage sharing and discussion at many levels. I am acutely aware that this book is, for me, also shaped by a Western-centric and, in particular, a UK- and USA-centric focus, which is made even narrower by my ability to share only my own personal and professional experiences and learning of this vast topic. We need only look to our European neighbours to experience very different approaches and attitudes to sex and older adults. My experience of older adults in Italy, especially, is that many will meet daily to drink an espresso at the bar, dressed and groomed to the hilt, to gossip, flirt extravagantly and then go home. If they happen to meet one another in the street, they will engage in a round of flirting and joking that makes the outsider (me!) blush. Full of caffeine, verve and wellbeing, they have asserted themselves as still fun-loving and viable sexual beings, even if they return home to their spouse of 60 years, their extended family or the dog. In other cultures, the rise of the senior living community and holidays and cruise ships dedicated to the over-60s – freed from societal constraints and expectations, and with cash to spare – has seen a rise in late-life leisure activities and enjoyment of all kinds, including sexual.

The broad range of human sexuality and its fulfilment can be as diverse and imaginative as the individuals on the planet, and in trying to be appropriate, even a non-binary designation of sexual preference – or one that I might imagine is inclusive – is still likely to be flawed and exclusive.

We need to challenge our beliefs that we are indeed sensitive and inclusive in our relationships and in the management of services and the training and supervision of our staff. It is not sufficient to be observant and vigilant about stereotyping, prejudice, ignorance and denial. Without our knowledge and sensitive awareness, individuals who differ from one another may be rendered invisible or not worthy of consideration and kindness and the upholding of their human rights. However, the process of raising awareness of diversity and equality begins with ourselves and the level of acceptance and knowledge we find within. Assumptions can too often be made about our openness and welcome of difference in all of its forms. There are some excellent checklists and recommendations made in the documents mentioned above. A particular favourite is Sally Knocker's Age UK publication *Safe to Be Me* (Knocker and Smith 2017) which has especially useful points for reflection and training.

It is in this little spoken of, yet hugely personal and motivational aspect of adult lives that we may find our biggest challenges, as it reflects and involves us all.

I am also only discussing here forms of sexual expression that are consensual and legal. As a therapist, I know that women's and men's sexual preferences, which bring them a sense of pleasure and ultimately 'wellbeing', are beyond the scope of this book. These men and women may also develop dementia, and in the forgetting and in their experience of disinhibition we may hear about or observe behaviour that has previously been private – as with most aspects of disinhibited language, thoughts and behaviour.

It was concerning to me, although not surprising, that professionals across the health and social care spectrum generally, including the counselling profession, were not always open or informed about sexuality in later life and certainly had not considered it as part of the lives of people living with dementia. The topic often resulted in prejudice and stereotyping, sometimes openly expressing shame, disgust or ridicule. And why wouldn't it be so? It would be a reflection of society at large. The most private and intimate of human behaviours pitches itself against the youth culture and the incest taboo, cultural values and spirituality as well as inherent ageist, racist and sexist stereotyping, homophobia and transphobia, and discrimination against those with disabilities or mental health challenges.

If you are living with dementia, this small offering may go some way to redress the balance and encourage you to believe in your right to be considered a sexual person if you so wish, irrespective of whether you choose to be sexually active or not. If you do, there might be a chance that someone outside your immediate circle will offer an opportunity for a helpful conversation, and perhaps together you might discover some practical and life-affirming alternatives and opportunities.

In the overall scheme of things, challenges around sexuality and living with dementia occur less often than we would imagine, and, in many cases, healthy and affirming sexual relationships are maintained or newly emerge. We may never hear of any sexual issues or concerns while men and women are able to live without the input of health and social care, with their privacy intact. Sex and relationships and/ *or* opportunities for sex usually only come to our attention when there are problems or concerns associated with them.

However, when difficulties do occur, there is often a charged atmosphere, embarrassment, misunderstanding, feelings of anger and shame, accusations and involvement of safeguarding teams, social workers, partners, families and sometimes media reporting. Knowledge, awareness, training, sensitivity and practical solutions for all concerned can go a long way to prevent most upsetting situations and support the quality of life that does not make sex invisible or a problem to 'deal with' only when challenges occur.

In writing this book, I am drawing on nearly 40 years of experience in both the USA and UK as a nurse and specialist in dementia care working with persons living with dementia and their partners, carers, families and the professionals who support them. As a counsellor, I have been privileged to hear the sexual concerns, successes, loss, trauma and new-found delight of numerous men and women. I have been involved in developing and delivering training around issues of sexuality, ageing and dementia. We have learned a great deal over the years, and many professionals have transformed how they, their staff and their clients benefit from innovative and sensitive insights and support around sex. Yet there is always more for us all to learn.

The other perspective is from my own counselling relationships with men and women living with dementia from age 39 to 85, and from counselling carers who spoke about changes in their sex lives since the diagnosis of dementia in their partner. Occasionally, the client would be an adult child or other relative who was the mistaken object of affection or overtly sexualised comments and behaviour. More often than not, they would have been contacted to discuss what to do about Aunt Joan or Cousin Tony, Mum or Granddad's inappropriate sexual behaviour. Additionally, I have been called to consult with staff in a range of care environments about what they considered to be 'inappropriate sexual behaviour' and the challenges staff and families were facing. An open, informed and respectful attitude towards this most intimate behaviour, which can so suddenly become shared without the person's awareness or other people's consent, is essential as we support human rights and affirm identity, dignity, choice and control.

My first article about sex and older people was published in 2001 in *Signpost: Journal of Dementia and Mental Health Care of Older People* (Whitsed-Lipinska 2001), and later, with John Killick (2003), 'Sexually Speaking' as a contribution to *Pathways*, the newsletter of the Dementia Services Development Centre at Stirling University. This has required many hours of my own study, reflections, supervision and writing.

I was encouraged by many, but especially Dr Carole Archibald, to whom I owe a debt of gratitude for her early writing with clarity and inspiration on the topic of sex and dementia. I knew that I was on the right track. There were years of training health and social care professionals begun in New Hampshire, USA, in the early 1980s in the hope that by sharing experiences we might create together a new paradigm that truly involves and respects the whole person.

There are, however, many instances in my experience when the issues of sexual identity and expression, appropriate discussions, actions and support have given me reason to rejoice and be hopeful. I know that we can sometimes do this well and that we are learning with one another as we live out our intentions as loving and caring inclusive human beings to be even more helpful and helpful more often.

But the biggest barriers and obstacles may often be our own internal conversations, thoughts, beliefs and fears. When we can get past these, we can celebrate together the joy and comfort and often passionate relationships for those of us fortunate enough to have them in whatever stage or state of life. We can encourage others to become more open and flexible and non-judgemental towards one another as we age or live with dementia.

What I am proposing in this book is the opportunity to view adult sexuality in its beauty, expansiveness and complexity as a part of nurturing wellbeing when living with dementia.

This means, essentially, that we look at the flip side of this well-worn coin which has valuable and essential learning for us all and may not have been given much attention – the side of the coin that offers a positive outlook on sexuality and dementia. My dear friend and colleague, the Julian scholar, priest and therapist Robert Fruehwirth, offers us an approach that I believe is also fitting here. He invites us to imagine holding two possibly conflicting voices in the same room of our minds, respecting both, being attuned to both without judgement. In that spirit, knowing what we know about sexual vulnerability, being mindful of past trauma, the need to prevent harm and abuse, to celebrate difference and desire, we can also give equal voice and place to sex and intimacy in the lives of men and women living with dementia, and its contribution towards wellbeing. I can hold both of these conversations in my mind and spirit. I invite you to do the same. Initially, it may feel somewhat strange, but, as with most things, practice may help us create a new focus, open and creative thinking and feeling about a special area of our shared humanity and what happens to it and us when our brain changes.

Who knows where this may lead? I hope you feel encouraged to ask your questions honestly of yourself, and sometimes of others, and have those conversations for the first time or maybe the umpteenth time. Perhaps we might not find the answers yet, but staying open to the questions invites openness and that allows room for the creative and the spiritual.

I have felt a real sense of privilege and gratitude in welcoming the generous narratives of persons living with dementia, so that we can hear their voices and read their narratives in this book.

I have made every effort to disguise, make anonymous and consolidate the real experiences and conversations of clients, relatives and staff without losing the essential point of their experience. Yet you may feel as though this is your own experience or that of a family or staff member. This only serves to highlight the experiences that are often consistent within the lives of those living with dementia or supporting others. Some of the narratives are of women and men no longer living. You may recognise some aspects of the narratives from other published articles or books of mine. If they have had a particular relevance to this topic, I may have renamed the person or reframed the content to make more sense here.

My hope is that this important aspect of Self is embraced, respected and included when thinking about and supporting men and women living with dementia, whether single or in partnership and across the great variety of sexual experiences that exist. I also hope that relatives and friends and the professionals who support them may also find interest here.

This small offering is my own limited overview to the background we all share. It is also an attempt to outline the starting point for discussions for some and to affirm current developments and best practice for others.

I hope that we can continue to improve quality of life for those living with dementia, particularly by including a closer look at sexuality.

For all of my limitations, I apologise in advance.

What to Expect

The style of writing in this book is deliberately non-academic and, I hope, easy to read for anyone who is interested. There are many more erudite and thorough texts written about living with dementia, about wellbeing, about sex and dementia, and about ageing and dementia. I would not wish to compete with them. I have yet to find one with a title and approach like this one. Rather, I would prefer you find in these pages ways to stimulate your own development, create discussion, enhance relationships and think new thoughts. Perhaps what is written will encourage your current outlook and beliefs and affirm your already good professional practice.

Chapter 1 introduces the subject within the present context of the topics of wellbeing, sex, sex and older adults, and sex and living with dementia and living with difference, in particular cultural and LGBTQI difference. The need for mental capacity and consent around sexual situations is also explored.

Chapter 2 explores biology and the 'biological imperatives' or 'must do' list of human survival and where sex fits in. The brain and dementia and the brain and sex will be discussed. Mention will be made of the brain and embodied cognition, and how it is affected by changes associated with dementia, which in turn affects behaviour, intimacy and attachment.

Chapter 3 will offer a brief review of the need for sensuality, sexuality and intimacy and the frequent challenges that emerge. It will include an exploration of relationships with family, lovers and friends, the environment and sex, misunderstanding and miscuing in the area of sensuality, sexuality and intimacy, and focus on person-centred conversations and a holistic approach including the development of a person-centred sexual profile based on Kitwood's psychological needs of people with dementia.

Chapter 4 briefly examines Carl Rogers' and Tom Kitwood's contributions to the person-centred approach and how that has had an impact on supporting people living with dementia. It describes responses to sensuality, sex, spirituality and living well with dementia. Kitwood's psychological needs of persons with dementia will be discussed within a sexual context, helping us to create guidelines for person-centred conversations that could lead to creating a person-centred sexual profile for an individual.

Chapter 5 includes training tools to enhance our understanding and appreciation of sex, dementia and wellbeing, with suggestions for moving forward. In this process, I hope that the reader will have reviewed their own views about sex and considered areas that may cause them to question their openness, and consider aspects they might find challenging as well as using materials to support training.

1

Dementia and Wellbeing

Over many years and many relationships with women and men living with dementia, I have come to appreciate that individual responses to living with dementia are numerous, varied and often surprising. I remember one gentleman telling me that his daughter's concern for his wellbeing was causing him grief. It was more alarming to him than his new diagnosis of Alzheimer's disease. He wanted to maintain his routine of getting on the double-decker bus (the old London Routemaster variety with an open platform at the back) into town to get his newspaper and look around the shops before coming home again for his lunch. His daughter was concerned that he might fall off the back of the bus and be injured or worse, or forget how to get home at all. 'If I fall off, I fall off. It won't be because I have Alzheimer's. If I forget where I am, someone will help me. I want to live my life to death.' He reluctantly agreed to carry an identity card in his wallet and have a label sewn into his favourite cap. He was less likely to lose his cap than his wallet. But he held on to what gave him a sense of identity and wellbeing. That, for him, was being able to continue with his routine for as long as possible. His daughter's sense of wellbeing, however, was only marginally improved. What brings each of us a sense of wellbeing is unique and incredibly important. One size does not fit all, yet our appreciation of the kinds of things that may create wellbeing in humans can assist us in finding the key to a given individual's preferences. The experiences of sex, intimacy, affection and sensuality are known to increase feelings of wellbeing. That does not mean to say that the absence of them in our lives means that we do not experience wellbeing at all. We know, of course, that this is not the case. The point of this book, after all, is to explore the idea that if these are areas of a person's life that they enjoyed prior to developing dementia, then how do we maintain those aspects of meaningful living? If living with dementia now opens a door to previously unexpressed or unexperienced and newly emerging aspects of Self, then how do we, in person-centred ways, support the needs and rights of the individual while, at the same time, ensuring their safety and dignity and that of others? These are the questions I hope this book will inspire you to address.

Wellbeing will be explored here in relation to living with dementia as it was first described at Bradford University with Tom Kitwood at the helm. We will explore the development of the person-centred approach in the work of Carl Rogers, which was the foundation of Kitwood's writings. We will introduce sex in later life, sex and dementia, and living with difference and how that affects who we are as sexual people.

We have long been indebted to the seminal work of Tom Kitwood (1997) and others in introducing us to the concepts of personhood and wellbeing in living with dementia. His research and writings from the early 1990s, with Kathy Bredin and others and, later, Professor Dawn Brooker's VIPS[1] (2006)

1　V = Valuing the person with dementia and those who care for them; I = treating people as Individuals; P = looking at the world from the Perspective of the person with dementia; S = a positive Social environment in which the person living with dementia can experience wellbeing.

approach have been transformational. More recently, Dr Caroline Baker's book *Developing Excellent Care for People Living with Dementia in Care Homes* (2015) highlighting the PEARL (Positively Enriching And enhancing Residents' Lives) model of caring in care homes, has informed and inspired the ways in which we create and sustain relationships with persons living with dementia and how we conceptualise and carry out their care. The journals and bookshelves are filled with variations on Kitwood's themes, which have proved vital to the collective and individual growth of our understanding and compassion. The practice of Dementia Care Mapping, with its checklists of illbeing and wellbeing indicators, was created in response partly to the pervasive state of illbeing which was then the status quo. Its widespread use and success has been the best way we know so far by which behaviour of the person living with dementia and the interactions with staff in the care home have become part of a systematic, evidence-based practice. The process then can inform improvements in care practice, which it is hoped will result in more frequent and consistent experiences of wellbeing for the person living with dementia and a sense of worth and achievement for the staff member. A very appealing combination, which has and continues to have broad appeal and particular benefits that have been evaluated elsewhere.

Years later, we can find ourselves overwhelmed by the well-intentioned idea of what it means to be 'person-centred' and find that in many situations it has lost its original intent and meaning. One can seek for indicators of wellbeing to the detriment of the person's right to simply 'be'. The idea of wellbeing is a particularly unique state which may have some general threads, most of which would serve to identify that the state being experienced was not illbeing – so therefore it must be wellbeing. I wonder if there is perhaps an in-between state, called simply 'being', which may represent a person's right to not feel particularly well or ill? They just *are*, in a neutral state of being OK with the present moment. Our pursuit of wellbeing could also lead us into trouble by limiting the vast human range of experience and reducing it to what a textbook or a zealous care worker might interpret as how a person living with dementia *ought* to be experiencing the moment. If I was to ignore the appropriate feeling just because it was not 'wellbeing', I could demean, dismiss and disempower the individual in question. I feel it would perhaps serve us better to return again and again, moment by new moment, to the unique 'perceptual field' of the individual that Rogers describes in Number 2 of his 19 Propositions (1951). He says essentially that the individual will react to what is around her as it is experienced and perceived, processed and understood. This perceptual field then becomes 'reality' to the individual. In relationship with that other person, I can feel and hear and sense their current level of experiencing. They can also place me in that present moment, within their reality. This is at the heart of the person-centred approach with which Tom Kitwood would have been especially familiar.

This attuned relationship approach is also currently at the heart of the work developed by Susanna Howard and Living Words in the UK (2014). Howard and her colleagues create relationships with persons living with dementia in care homes and through that relationship observe their state of being and hear their words, creating unique poetry which is shared with the person with dementia, their families and the staff who support them. The results are poignant and remarkable reminders of the individual who remains with us, but because of confusion of language or absence of language may be overlooked or rendered invisible or of little note.

One could argue that what these women and men living with often advanced dementia experience is a real sense of wellbeing, as do all those connected with the project. Staff in particular are often awakened to a different way of relating to the resident and learn new ways of interacting based on the training they are part of during the project. Taking part in a meaningful and life-enhancing activity together is likely to improve the wellbeing of all concerned.

The Oxford Dictionary defines wellbeing as 'the state of being comfortable, healthy or happy'. As you can imagine, this covers a great deal of territory for any individual. Then there is the wellbeing of the group to consider. In my experience, it is often the coming together of the needs and wants of the individual, as they affect the group or are affected by the group, where tensions and challenges may occur when sex, intimacy and relationships are the theme. The 'group' may initially be the person's family group, their social group, their own living community including clubs, pubs, restaurants, places of worship and so forth. As mainly social creatures who value the approval of and inclusion within the group, it is not always easy for us to swim against the tide, do our own thing and thumb our noses at the established 'norms'. Finding and maintaining a balance in an ever-changing population with ever-changing and unique needs is a mammoth task. I have observed and heard about excellent practice over the years and in many different locations that is a living testimony to the flexibility, determination, expertise and compassion of women and men in various roles and communal environments. We are only too familiar with the occasions when this doesn't work well, and certainly there is yet much for us to do together to improve standards and expectations for living well with dementia. However, this is an opportunity to highlight the actual or potential positive experiences and to celebrate what is working well. This could also mean that sex is not a part of a person's life at all. That is fine. My focus is on those people for whom no one has imagined that the presence or absence of sex or sexuality is part of their story, whether they have been sexually active or not in their lifetime.

Sex and Later Life

We are living with two generations of people and their sexual histories. In terms of living with dementia, it would be a mistake to imagine that women and men between the ages of 40 (or younger) and 100-plus would share much in common in terms of their sexual histories. Let's look briefly at the changes in support group participants as an indicator of historical changes in my own work in family support groups over two continents and 30 years. A typical support group in the 1980s was comprised mainly of family caregivers, mostly spouses, and adult sons and daughters, brothers and sisters or an occasional friend. By the 1990s a 'typical' group had evolved into a couple of spouses, a life-long unmarried lesbian partner, a man in his late 80s caring for his son with *HIV/ AIDS*-related dementia, a 15-year-old granddaughter who was caring for her grandmother with advanced Alzheimer's disease, and her mother who was an alcoholic with severe mental health concerns, all in the same house. This combination of relationships happens more frequently than we might imagine and often also includes grandchildren and great-grandchildren, sometimes all sharing the same house. Who has the time or energy or privacy for sex in this not-uncommon scenario? As we know only too well, challenges to sexual desire and behaviour also emerge as part of a pattern of normal ageing and along the adult developmental continuum. When a person receives a diagnosis of dementia, then all of the 'givens' of these intricate relationships and the balancing of independent and interdependent lives will be reorganised and recreated. Often this experience has been helpful in making decisions about what a person really wants from life, what or who they find they no longer wish to live with or spend time with. They can discuss how much they can 'pare down' to the minimum for a good and healthy life, with less 'clutter' of the emotional and physical kind. The less the brain has to struggle with, the better. This leaves space and energy for the really important and essential people, places and events in life that a person does not want to limit or exclude. It can also mean letting go of so much that we think we need to have around us in order to function well. Those all-important standards that we impose on ourselves and that others impose on us do not seem to hold the same significance. Being able to simplify life and the living of it has been described by many people living with dementia and those who love and support them as unexpected gifts.

We had wanted to get rid of so many things for a long time and now we finally had good reason to do so. Limiting the number of choices Gwen had to make over every aspect of her day was distressing and, quite frankly, unnecessary. It really frustrated her and drove me mad with impatience. Kitchen drawers contained only the essentials and one of everything else, not four types of the same thing. I had dishes in reserve for when family or friends came round to eat with us, but the cabinets had only our two of each thing for us. Dining items, clothing and shoes were taken to charity shops or re-housed in the spare room for when she needed something particular. Make-up and toiletries were cut back to only one of each item, but with the spares elsewhere. We have a favourite café that we have been going to for years, for coffee or lunch or afternoon tea. They always have a very attractive table setting, but, for Gwen, that meant more clutter and more choices, more distraction and irritation for us both. We have known them there for so long that I felt quite happy calling ahead and letting them know we were coming in and asking for our favourite table. There was one knife and fork, one spoon, a mug for each of us, a salt shaker only. Other condiments could be asked for as needed. If we wanted water as well, the glass of water would arrive on its own. We sit over by the window and out of the direct busy flow of the café. We have been able to continue our pleasure of going out to eat together and will continue to do so, even though it's not quite as often as it used to be.

This experience greatly adds to the sense of wellbeing that is important for Gwen and Martin as a couple and enhances their opportunities for being out, planning ahead and involving others to support them to continue living well with dementia.

It is true for many persons living with dementia and their partners and family that friends and loved ones seem to disappear, and people often experience real feelings of loss, grief, rejection, isolation, anger, loneliness and resulting depression. For many others, friends and family really step up and make every effort to continue with adjusting and adapting to a relationship with new aspects of the Self now living with dementia. This requires an open heart and mind and a willingness to listen to what the person living with dementia senses is important in the relationship and in their lives.

A recent study entitled 'Sexual health and wellbeing among older men and women in England' from the University of Manchester (2016) is the first of its kind to include participants in their 80s. Dr David Lee reports: 'Our ongoing research is also highlighting the diversity of late-life sexualities and trying to impose youthful norms of sexual health on older people would be over-simplistic and even unhelpful' (p.45). How essential it is to know that comparisons are no longer relevant to a group that one no longer belongs to. To even the score, older people are deciding what their sexuality is and is not, and are talking about it.

Yet assumptions are often made – and we can completely miss the influences history has had on the sex lives of persons living with dementia – and may become part of an invisible narrative that it would be important to explore. For example, a care worker might find it odd that Jerry Bright, who he suspects is gay, is not 'out'. 'In this day and age, why ever not!' he replied when told that Jerry wanted to keep this aspect of his life private, but wanted the staff to be aware. Jerry and his friends remembered well what it was like to be gay and living with the possibility that if you came out, or were 'outed', you could be imprisoned. He knew of others and had himself been taunted, beaten, ridiculed and abused. He had friends who had lost their careers, their families, friends and their children. That exploration in history may not always be with the person themselves, but it will benefit our own education and enlightenment and awareness. Knowing some of the backdrop to our clients' emerging sexuality and their adult development can give us great insight into who the person is now, and how we might best support them. A reminiscence group, for Jerry, for example, may not be the most comfortable of events.

In her recent book *Scary Old Sex* (2016), Arlene Heyman creates delicious and poignant stories of sex in later life in ways that may seem shocking to some. And yet, by the standards of similar literature, it is fairly restrained. But it is beautifully honest, wrinkles and all. Years ago, I remember being delighted and intrigued by Jane Juska's ground-breaking true story, *A Round-Heeled Woman: My Late-Life Adventures in Sex and Romance* (2004, p.12), from which comes the memorable quote: 'Before I turn 67 next March, I would like to have a lot of sex with a man I like.' So began her advertisement in the *New York Times*, and her escapades became the theme of her book which is bold and enlightening and very entertaining.

In her bestseller *Prime Time: Love, Health, Sex, Fitness, Friendship, Spirit – Making the Most of All Your Life* (2012), Jane Fonda writes about sex and older people in general, and also about her own sex life in the later years and how surprised she has been by its evolution.

Erica Jong, who has seen most of a particular generation through their coming of age, continues her own coming-of-age narrative in *Fear of Dying* (2015), which, of course, includes her musings and escapades into sex in later life while grieving over the loss of her ardent husband due to illness. Her daughter is about to have her first child. At the same time, she is caring for and despairing over her very elderly parents who are both physically and cognitively frail.

There are also more roles than ever before in television drama, in theatre and in film for older people and sexual relationships or sexual situations. Most recent of these concerning a person living with dementia was the film *Still Alice* (2014) starring Julianne Moore in an Oscar-winning performance. It was gratifying to see the whole of her character as the rare form of familial Alzheimer's disease progressed, including her sexual self.

I am reminded of a particularly beautiful passage in a favourite book, *The Notebook* by Nicholas Sparks, written in 1996, which I read in one leap across the ocean on a flight from London to Boston, crying most of the way. In the section I refer to, the long-lost lovers are reunited but now in a care home. Allie has Alzheimer's disease, and she and Noah become lost in one another again as they rediscover their passion and tenderness.

Neither age nor dementia can stop our quest for love, romance, intimacy and sexual connection if the desire is still with us. That, of course, can be both a blessing and a curse. Most of the time, it just *is*. I believe our role is to bring this often private and silent part of us in line with other aspects of Self and identity which we profess to uphold.

The LGBTQI community is also part of the context of 21st-century literature, film and television, but my experience of this genre is limited. My awareness of the protagonists also living with dementia is even more limited.

The 'baby boomers' who were part of the sexual revolution, women's lib and the pill and enjoyed 'free love' unfettered by social convention, often disinhibited by drugs and/or alcohol, music and communal living, may now be those being diagnosed with dementia. We would wish to offer an openness of regard and contextual appreciation for their sexual histories and expectations in later life that may be very different to our own expectations. Is it possible that, given cognitive changes, they may perceive the residential home as a 'commune' similar to the ones that they lived and loved in?

Our elders of the next round are also those who may have had flourishing careers with large salaries and entertainment involving sex – with alcohol, recreational drugs, 'legal highs' as well as cocaine and combinations of drugs and alcohol to induce sexual edge. It would be advisable to have conversations about these potential issues before we find ourselves wondering how to respond most appropriately.

Living with Difference

Our ageing selves become more and more the invisible members of Western society, except when we are told how much of a burden we are and how much we are costing everyone else to stay alive. When our physical and mental health begins to deteriorate, and creates a challenge to ourselves, our families and society at large, the older generations, grandparents and great-grandparents, may begin to doubt their place in society, that they ever mattered and that their lives are testimonies to their tenacity, creativity and resilience. The invisibility that comes with ageing is no respecter of gender, culture or sexual preference. It is made more difficult in groups where prejudice and stereotyping have already rendered individuals invisible as well as disenfranchised, often outside their own family groups and culture.

We are all living with difference – how that is experienced will depend on our gender, culture, birth-place, education, upbringing, values, faith, economics and politics, where we find ourselves living and with and among whom. The LGBTQI community may find themselves more misunderstood, more invisible, especially as they age. We know that more older LGBTQI people are single, live alone and have fewer involved relatives or children. A study by the New York Brookdale Center for Healthy Aging, quoted by Sally Knocker in *Safe to Be Me* (Knocker and Smith 2017), bears this out and states that there are likely to be higher numbers of LGBTQI people living in care homes than we expect. The study found that, compared with the heterosexual population, LGBTQI people were two times more likely to be single, two and a half times more likely to live alone and four and a half times more likely to have no children. Living with dementia may also mean that after years of living in ways expected of them both culturally and socially, women and men may find a way to live as their authentic and non-heterosexual selves at last.

Women are also living with difference in terms of both living with dementia themselves and caring for others who have dementia. In a recent, illuminating and important study, 'Women and Dementia: A Global Research Review' (Erol, Brooker and Peel 2015), with Alzheimer's Disease International, Professor Dawn Brooker and associates conducted a review of the research literature to date. Their findings show us not only that there are more women than men living with dementia, but also that they are the primary caregivers in the healthcare setting and at home, and that they are those who have the least income and the greatest need to work. No wonder they also report feeling more burdened by their roles. I have known women who have been nurses and healthcare assistants, who go home after a long and demanding day to care for a parent living with dementia at home with them and their teenage children, and who then develop a dementia in later life themselves. These concerning and important data also have an implication for women and sex. Some of us may be simply too exhausted to be interested in sex, alone or with another. Others may be very keen to exit the workaday travails that have befallen us and look forward to momentary bliss and escape.

A recent online article from the *Telegraph* (Sawer 2017) interviews Patricia Davis, born Peter, a retired WWII soldier and loving husband of 63 years. She claims she had known she was in the wrong body from the age of three. She learned about herself through a *television programme*. She learned that she was not alone, that her experiences were shared by others and that they had a name: transgender. She told her wife, who was very supportive, before she died, but they decided to keep it secret. Now, at age 90, Patricia is living as a woman, is undergoing transition treatment and is 'having a great time' and 'a new lease of life'.

We might assume that a person living with dementia at home as a single person, or with a partner, continues to enjoy their sex life with little or no changes, but we might be wrong. I have been told that for some people, as dementia progresses, changes consistent with depression, other forms of brain injury, learning and physical disabilities occur. These changes alter sexual desire, functioning, performance and enjoyment. These changes can be consistent with age or, with younger-onset dementia, more consistent with changes in brain function. This will have a direct effect on the individual and any possible partner(s). I will refer to this in more detail in a later chapter.

Marjorie was a retired teacher who spent many happy years in the local amateur dramatics society and played the organ at her church. She had been married for 35 years when her husband died. Marjorie had loving relationships with her three children and five grandchildren. She loved to travel and play tennis. She developed young-onset dementia and eventually it was unsafe for her to stay in her home even with support. She was living in sheltered accommodation where she enjoyed singing her favourite musical songs to anyone she found in the lounge. She declared with great joy and enthusiasm that she was finally free, and she was going to live the rest of her life as a lesbian, which she said she had always been. This was met with mixed responses from her family and friends, including shock and anger, disbelief, indifference, celebration and support.

A newly emerging and less inhibited Marjorie was taking a courageous leap towards a more authentic life, actually encouraged by her age and diagnosis.

In multicultural Britain, people living with dementia include an ageing refugee population and newly arrived immigrants with their own sexual values, customs and traditions, including what does and does not constitute criminal sexual behaviour in the UK. At times our desire to understand, appreciate and support individuals and communities may be at odds with human rights and the law, which can create further challenges. Willingness to be open to the situation and supportive of the human beings involved, while still upholding the law, may challenge the very fabric of our assumed rights, freedoms and privilege very deeply.

Many years ago I remember being invited to a care home to talk with staff and the family of an elderly Hindu lady with Alzheimer's disease. Her condition was making it impossible to be cared for by her family at home, which was devastating to the family, and placement in the care home was seen as a great failure and cultural affront.

Mrs Patel had formed an affectionate and caring (non-sexual) relationship with a white male resident, Jim Smith. Both of their eyes lit up when they saw one another, and they would go for long walks around the grounds, sit in the garden and eat meals together. They were always holding hands and chatting endlessly. Staff were not sure what they were chatting about, but they both seemed to be engaged, animated and happy. Sometimes they would sit together in either of their rooms and would enjoy having their afternoon tea there together. Although this may seem at first like a mutually enhancing scenario of wellbeing, you can perhaps imagine that the extended family of Mrs Patel was not happy with this situation at all. The staff were informed by the eldest son that they would have to move Mr Smith if 'it isn't stopped':

> Our mother has been a widow for 16 years. She will not have looked at another man since our father died. She knows this. She would not wish to. And he is not even of our own culture. How could you all have allowed this to develop? This is just terrible. You should know better than to allow this.

It was difficult to see the family so distressed. The staff wanted to maintain the good relationship they already had and show their genuine concern for their feelings and respect for their culture. Mr Smith's family was more than happy with the situation: 'It's the first time Dad's been happy since he came here.'

The first consideration was for Mrs Patel, Mr Smith and their apparent wishes and wellbeing.

In this scenario, we can see the difficulty of adult children acknowledging their parent as capable of intimacy and relationship needs with members of the opposite sex. We also witness the important cultural and traditional norms and expectations thwarted by the effects of dementia. We *learn* how to behave in our families, our cultures, our faith. We rely on *memory* to help us keep up with the expectations that learned behaviour has instilled. Mrs Patel's extended family came to a meeting at the care home. Because of the rapport that had previously existed between the staff and the family, there was a great deal of good will involved in the discussions amidst the disappointment and anger. Deep feelings were expressed by the family and compassionate listening skills employed by the care home staff. Once the role of dementia and memory and culture and faith had been explored, and the obvious benefits to Mrs Patel examined, it was decided that Mrs Patel could continue her friendship with Mr Smith as long as it remained platonic and beneficial to Mrs Patel. It was agreed that Mrs Patel would have special time with her family when Mr Smith was otherwise occupied. Sometimes Mrs Patel would be taken with family to the local park and to a nearby café where she had always enjoyed socialising with her friends.

Sex, Dementia and Wellbeing

If we talk about holistic, inclusive and person-centred support of men and women living with dementia, it is essential that we include in our conversations with them what is changing in their lives from the perspective of their relationships, sexual and otherwise (including pets and social media friends), their ability for fun and stress reduction and their spirituality if they have one. Although the functional changes associated with memory loss are complex and often difficult to navigate, we seem to have those conversations and propose solutions to them more readily than those of a relational, sexual, sensual nature.

Too often, particularly within the culture at large and the realm of adult services across the spectrum, issues of sexuality as part of identity and human rights and an indicator of healthy adult status and wellbeing are ignored.

Of course, anyone over 40 will be well aware of how the goalposts keep moving regarding ageing in our society: 60 is the new 50 and on it goes... And our teenage children and grandchildren often see us as definitely uncool and clearly disgusting if anything to do with sex or romance is mentioned to do with their parents.

The incest taboo exists for a reason and, in the West, it is a criminal offence to cross those established lines. However, the same criteria designed to keep children sexually safe within a family and a society and free from exploitation also contribute to the challenge adult children face when encountering their parents' and grandparents' rights to privacy and sexual expression. When those adults are also living with dementia, the adult children and grandchildren often find it awkward and difficult – if not impossible – to view that relative with objectivity, realism, compassion and human rights when it comes to sex and relationships.

Often this is where a trusted professional or best friend can be the one to have conversations the 'children' cannot and maybe would do well to avoid in order to allow some modicum of control and privacy for all concerned.

One evening, Alice comes to see her mother Gill at the care home. The door to her bedroom is closed, and Alice can hear that she is not alone.

Without knocking, Alice throws open the door to find Eddie, another resident, and Gill in Gill's bed, and she could see that they were kissing. 'What on earth are you doing in here? This is disgusting behaviour!' The couple looked shocked and embarrassed and sat up quickly. Gill says to Eddie, 'It's all right. Stay here.' Alice becomes more angry and agitated and grabs Eddie to get him out of the bed. She pulls the alarm buzzer. 'You get back to your room, you dirty old man. You stay away from my mother.' When Sally, the staff member, arrives, hearing the shouting, Alice is already getting out her mobile phone. 'How can you let my mother be assaulted like this! I brought her here for care and look what has happened. I'm going to call the police.'

Although Alice's reaction is understandable, there are many ways in which this might have been prevented and the privacy and dignity of the couple upheld. Imagine, in particular, how Eddie might have been feeling. Gill sounded as if she didn't want him to leave – how might she be feeling? Could a conversation with Alice about changes to relationships and sexual needs and feelings have been helpful before her mother came to live at the care home?

In particular, this conversation could have explored how they might all respond should Gill wish to be in a relationship, either platonic or sexual, with another resident. Issues concerning capacity and safeguarding will have to be raised and appropriate documentation and directives put in place. The important questions of rights and freedom versus vulnerability will need to be discussed and agreed upon in the best interests of Gill and Eddie, rather than their families. Alice will need support and reassurance and an opportunity to be heard. However, Alice's reactions and responses, important as they are, are more in keeping with the challenge of adult children seeing their aged parents living with dementia as having any vestiges of sexual feelings and behaviours ever, and especially now.

Over time and with some hesitation, Alice could see that her mother and Eddie were enjoying one another's company. She got to know Eddie's family who were content with the situation and helped her to see the value of the relationship for as long as they were both happy.

The issues of mental capacity and consent are at the forefront of our desire to safeguard men and women 'at risk'. I refer the reader to the Mental Capacity Act (2005) which describes the details of capacity. However, the first and most important principle is that all people are considered to have capacity until proven otherwise. The Deprivation of Liberty Safeguards (DoLS) (2009) is an amendment to that Act in order to ensure that we are acting in a person's 'best interest'. In unusual circumstances, where sexual obsession and harassment of individuals occurs, it may require specific ways to keep individuals in hospitals, care homes and institutions safe, and a DoLS application may need to be made. Issues of sexuality and self-expression are also contained within the principles of the Human Rights Act. Each individual's rights and needs should be assessed on an individual basis so that we do not make assumptions that could be false and damaging.

It is paramount that vulnerable women and men are not led into or left in harm's way and that every care is taken to prevent abuse and respond immediately to suspected or actual events.

In addition, we are also in the grip of two deeply ingrained prejudices: against old age and dementia. It is therefore imperative that we attempt to separate the events and status quo from stereotype and discrimination – our own and that of our wider society.

In its most subtle form, discrimination is hidden within the invisibility of sex in the lives of older people and people living with dementia.

Over the many years I have listened to older people's experiences as a counsellor, it seems that I have created a trusting relationship resulting in what I think is a fairly unusual determination in the client. It emerges over time. Inevitably, by the third session, the client would have voluntarily told me the details of their sex lives past and present and often their hopes for the future. From the very frank, detailed, sometimes poignant, often romantic, tragic or traumatic sharing, their narrative showed that it was important to the person that I know these aspects of themselves.

I learned quickly not to make assumptions about the client's sexuality based on appearance, ability, diagnosis or living situation.

Phil was a successful retired car salesman referred to me for counselling as he was quite depressed following a moderate stroke and had recently been diagnosed with vascular dementia.

He had been married to Marilyn, his high school sweetheart, for 58 years and was hoping to celebrate their diamond wedding anniversary. By session three, it seemed that Phil had found his courage and trusted me enough to begin by saying:

P: It's about the sex. That's why I'm so depressed.

D: You think that's what's making you feel depressed, Phil?

P: Now I've had this stroke, and my memory is going, I have a stick and a wheelchair to get around, I'm afraid I'm never going to do it again, you know...

D: You're afraid you won't be able to have sex with Marilyn again?

P: Yeah, but it's not like this is new; we haven't had it for years. And years. She kinda shut up shop after the change. One of the reasons I married young was to be able to have sex all the time with this gorgeous girl. Most of the time it's been great, then not so good when the kids were small. Then when the last one went off to college, it got better again. So it was a shock when she started putting me off, making excuses. She had always enjoyed it.

He went on to describe feeling frustrated, angry, depressed and resentful for more than 20 years, with only rare occasions of intimacy. Nor did they talk about what was no longer happening in the bedroom.

His strong faith helped him through, but also made him feel 'sinful' on rare occasions when he 'gave in to masturbation or die'. He saw this as the 'last resort', leaving him feeling 'guilty, dirty and a failure'.

Over the ensuing weeks of therapy, Phil decided that he wanted to work towards courting his wife and having sex at least one more time with his life-long lover before either his stroke or his dementia made it impossible, or he died.

Phil used the sessions to develop a plan of action, reporting at the next session on the outcomes and how he and his wife felt about what was happening. It was a gradual process of creating opportunities for closeness, touch, affection, kissing – none of which Marilyn resisted and indeed seemed to welcome. They began sitting together on the sofa to watch television rather than in two recliner chairs. Phil described wrapping his arms around his wife from behind as she washed the dishes and nuzzling her neck. This made them both laugh and joke, which led to more playfulness and intimacy.

One afternoon Phil arrived for our session grinning from ear to ear, and when he sat down, gave me a double thumbs-up. 'Twice!' he exclaimed.

He joyfully related how wonderful it had been for them both. He also expressed how grateful he was for having a chance to explore this area of his life, which, to date, no one had been willing to explore with him, including Marilyn.

Phil did not arrive for his planned session two weeks later. The social worker who had referred him called to say that Phil had died peacefully sitting out on his deck the previous week. I like to imagine he had a smile on his face. It is certainly a great testimony to the art of living in a state of wellbeing.

Unless you are a counsellor, you may be unlikely to hear these particular life stories. But as managers of services, health and social care professionals across the spectrum of care, you will also be having these conversations. However, it is not impossible, especially when supporting people with personal care where a sense of intimacy and safety may exist, that deep disclosures may emerge, and we need to be prepared. You may be just the right person at the right time. I concede that all of this requires our own self-evaluation, exploration of prejudices and a safe place to explore and challenge ourselves, whether in our own education, therapy or professional supervision. Our family and friends tend to support our own views, fears and ideas, so are not always the most helpful in these scenarios.

Angela Newman is the woman who taught me how to keep consent to sexual relating in perspective. She also taught me about deep and lasting love, and about compassion and passion as a means of communication with someone living with dementia. I have shared her story on numerous occasions with great effectiveness. I am so grateful not to have missed this particular lesson.

> The time had come for Peter to move to the local nursing home. He had moderate stage Alzheimer's disease, and Angela, his wife of 48 years, had cared for him in their home for the past seven of those years. There had been occasional extra support at home, and Peter had been to the care home for respite a few times, so that Angela could have a well-earned break. Now that her own health was deteriorating, and Peter's needs were increasing, she reluctantly decided that Peter had to move to the care home.
>
> Angela described how shocked and upset she was when she had asked for a double bed to be placed in Peter's room and was told that was not possible. Angela told the nurse that she and Peter had a close and loving relationship, and she wanted to be sure that they could continue this closeness as it was very important to them both.
>
> 'How would we know that your husband was consenting to any intimacy between you? His dementia is quite progressed now, which is why he is coming to live here after all.'

Although the concern for Peter is coming from a well-intentioned place, the attitude about it is one that is familiar and not very helpful or life-affirming.

Angela held her ground. She described how when she and Peter were intimate, when they made love, it didn't matter if he knew what day of the week it was, or who the president was, what his life's work had been, or his address. She wasn't sure he always knew her name, but he knew *her* in their intimacy. She also knew very clearly that he was 'consenting' to their intimacy and he would often initiate it and she was pleased to respond.

Angela reminded us all that, in a relationship of 48 years, sexual partners did not usually check with one another if they were consenting to sex. 'You just get to know one another's signals and body language.'

'Peter and I can really communicate without words. We really know one another in this private place. He remembers me. And us. It is what has kept me going and helped me to keep caring for him for the past seven years. Getting up again in the morning and doing the caregiver thing all over again was easier when I felt our love and closeness. I don't want us to lose each other just because he is moving house. I can't lose him twice. Not yet.'

Often the intimate connection is as much about the partner as it is for the person living with dementia. After this conversation, every effort was made to ensure that Angela and Peter had uninterrupted privacy and a double bed. Their relationship was respected and staff were considerate and supportive.

When the time came, Peter died in Angela's arms with their favourite classical music playing and soft lighting, alone, together, tucked up in their double bed.

The issues of consent and capacity are extremely important but they can be made more complex by our lack of understanding, openness and sensitivity. A person-centred approach will be our response to the individual people involved and their particular situation, and will respond to their feelings and needs as well as upholding safety and the law. Often as a result of fear within a 'blame culture', we go directly to the avoidance place in order to secure control and safety and to avoid 'getting it wrong' and triggering a safeguarding alert.

I highly recommend Luke Tanner's excellent chapter on 'Erotic Touch and Sexual Intimacy' in his book *Embracing Touch in Dementia Care: A Person-Centred Approach to Touch and Relationships* (2017). He helps us to explore the issue of 'erotic touch and touch to further intimacy' in ways that are open, frank and full of helpful examples taken from supporting people living with dementia in care environments.

It may be less easy to assess consent in a person with advanced dementia, but it will be obvious if the person is displaying signs of distress, anxiety, dislike or revulsion. We must be confident that dis-ease will be observable and we must respond immediately and involve partners and families in our discussions.

We walk the fine line between empowering independence and the right to self-expression and supporting 'at risk' vulnerable adults. However, when I have read some of the articles written on this topic designed to give guidance regarding consent to sexual engagement for people living with dementia in care facilities, I find that most items on the list of requirements would be hard to recognise in the normal to and fro of adult sexual engagement. There is also an assumption that thought and logic is a prerequisite for sex. Perhaps there exists in some an ability to plan for and regard the consequences of every sexual engagement, in which case those choices and activities would be informed. Living with dementia does not make our human heart and sexual desire any more capable of getting it right and making wise choices than when we live without it. Unfortunately, I have witnessed safeguarding alerts or police involvement in residential settings where neither would have happened if fear and panic had not created more difficulties. Having said that, it is of utmost importance that safeguarding policies and procedures are adhered to and that all is done to keep vulnerable men and women as safe as we are able. In the best sense, the safeguarding team is there to ensure safety of vulnerable and 'at risk' adults, but also to support and encourage best practice in the professionals involved. I feel it is important in our efforts to ensure safety that we do not create a double standard, the expectation of which most of us would find hard to meet.

Raising awareness and increasing our understanding, knowledge and sensitivity around issues of a sexual and sensual nature not only improve our relationships with those whom we support as professionals but adds to our sense of our own inner workings and paves the way for our own ageing selves and the event that we may develop dementia.

Introducing myself and others to the whole human person in a way that is respectful and aware that the person is also a sexual being (which also includes the need to define what that is for an individual, including being asexual) and possibly someone with a sexually active past, present and future helps to bring the whole person into focus.

Perhaps not in a malicious or intentional way, but almost more shocking is the pronouncement that 'the idea never crosses my mind', as one caregiver in a nursing home offered. Irrespective of whether we have conversations with individuals or not, if we do not entertain an awareness of the sexuality of that person on the grounds of ignorance or stereotyping and prejudice, we have actively discriminated against that person by rendering them invisible and not worthy of inclusion in our assessment of part of our humanity.

If we do have a conversation about sex and sexuality and what that means to a person, we may also gain an insight into areas of great pleasure, success, potency, sadness, grief, bitterness and hatred, love and romance. We may glimpse the divine and the spiritual, the thrill of the chase and the frisson of new romance – quite literally the bump and grind. We may hear about lovers won and lost and those never desired at all. Occasionally, conversations can lead to disclosures of abuse as either the victim or the perpetrator. I have encountered this during counselling sessions with older people who have not spoken about it for 70 years or more, but who have watched a recent television programme or seen a newspaper article which brought back memories, or allowed them for the first time to acknowledge their long-held secret and to put it into words and tears. Great care and sensitivity is needed to support women and men through this trauma; usually, the perpetrator(s) is no longer alive. A person may decide that you, in your role, are the person they wish to share this with. In moments of quiet and trust, or while having a manicure or a back rub, disclosures of this kind may occur. We need to be ever mindful that this may exist in the life history of any person living with dementia.

I have often been amazed when health, social care and counselling professionals who have attended my workshops and conference presentations, in spite of their many years of experience, their open and compassionate attitudes (often describing themselves as 'holistic' and 'person-centred' or 'relationship-centred') have said:

'It has never occurred to me before.'

'I haven't actually thought about this.'

'I don't need to know about this, it's never been an issue in our home.'

'I imagined it stopped being an issue once you were a certain age.'

'Oh, old people still do it, do they?'

'How can a person with Alzheimer's remember who she is having sex with, if she can't even remember her own name?'

'Vulnerable people need to be able to consent to sex – we can't have people just having sex with whoever they want whenever they want.'

You may recognise some of these statements having heard them from others or said them yourselves.

We may never be able to share the myriad diversity of sexualities that people now living with dementia embody. Being educated about equality and diversity and open and respectful of all human potentialities we bring our willingness to engage with the individual and unique person with all of their life experiences, including their sexuality. To profess to be truly person-centred and supporting men and women living with dementia in holistic ways, we need to be able to stretch ourselves and perhaps even venture out of our comfort zone in order to create comfort for another. We could make the assumption that while a person living with dementia at home, as a single person or with a partner, continues to enjoy their sex life with little or no changes, we might be wrong in some cases. I have been told that for some people, as dementia progresses, changes consistent with depression, other forms of brain injury, learning and physical disabilities occur. These changes alter sexual desire, functioning, performance and enjoyment. This will have a direct effect on the individual and any possible partner(s).

From the time of diagnosis, which could be as long as five years from the beginning of actual cognitive changes, there are likely to be physical and emotional changes that affect a person's interest in and abilities around sexual activity as with all other behaviours. That is a long time to be feeling awful about this aspect of your life and imagining your future with or without it, and not knowing who to talk to or where to look for information and support.

Because it is often believed that sex is private and a taboo subject, particularly if the client is the same age as your grandmother or your adult son, it is less likely than we might wish to be included in the assessments and questions evaluating behavioural change, either with the GP or the neurologist, old age psychiatrist or the memory clinic specialist. I remember seeing the box on an assessment form entitled 'Sexuality' and written in the box were the words 'wears lipstick'. What a missed opportunity!

And yet, most of the time, sex and its expression are addressed mainly from the perspective of disgust, fear and behaviours to be stopped and 'dealt with'. This often takes the form of accusations, safeguarding alerts or police involvement.

Although I appreciate there are indeed some dire situations that threaten individual rights and safety, this book will refer to these difficulties and challenges only briefly. We ignore our own and others' sexuality at our peril.

The peril is evident in the faces of those whose behaviour is misunderstood, in the open-mouthed horror of the untrained ingénue in the healthcare setting, the tears in the eyes of the abandoned lover.

It is not a mistake that a psychiatrist will ask a patient about the state of their libido or sex drive when making an assessment for depression. We do not feel like having sex when we can hardly get out of bed and brush our teeth. Adults who are well and healthy may choose to be engaged in sexual expression with another or alone. They may also choose to be celibate, either as a lifestyle choice or for a period of time. Celibacy can be overlooked as a valid choice in terms of one's sexuality and its expression. It may also be a reaction to a specific life situation such as a committed spiritual belief or way of life, loss of a partner through death, divorce or ongoing illness, or a time of healing from sexual trauma, to name but a few possibilities. Celibacy may become part of a loving sexual partnership 'for a season', agreed by both partners. It could be a 'time out' for a single person to focus on self-development, sport, academic or creative excellence, or simply to step off the treadmill of sexual expectations and pressures of the 21st century and contemplate their own sexuality.

Surely, our excellent care and support of persons with dementia may also result in the attributes of wellbeing.

Being in love and romantic intimacy are not only the domain of the young. However, the young often find it embarrassing to imagine their elders as sexual beings who may enjoy experiences similar to their own. Many of us are fortunate to find loving, romantic and passionate partnerships that last late into our lives. Later life can bring new-found opportunities for love, intimacy and passion. Age and diagnosis may not be a barrier to staying in love, or falling in love anew.

We are no strangers to the complexities and difficulties of finding and keeping love, and the complications of forbidden love. Our behaviours and desires are formed in the brain and body and create a complicated interweaving of neuronal impulses and production of chemicals which interact to give us our state of mind and emotion as well as our ability for the physical body to 'perform'. Our memory will also leap on to the scene with reminders of who we and our partner might be, past partners, trauma, the ways we enjoy or do not enjoy sex. A full-blown hidden or shared fantasy can operate at the same time as the lived experience of sex or even in its absence.

Dr Frans R. Hoogeveen, Associate Professor of Psycho-geriatrics at The Hague University of Applied Sciences, relates the content of his introductory lecture on ageing with students at the university. He shows a film which he describes as 'beautiful', 'well acted and tastefully filmed'. The couple making love on the floor of the man's apartment are in their 80s. He also shows still photographs of sexual intimacy between people in their 80s. The responses from the 20-year-olds is initially what we might predict – embarrassed giggling, then more raucous distaste. When asked if they would respond differently if the actors were beautiful and young, it was an emphatic 'yes'.

Hoogeveen writes:

Intimacy and sexuality are basic human needs that are intrinsic to people's sense of self and wellbeing. Regardless of age, individuals require companionship, intimacy and love, yet for older people this intrinsic right is often denied, ignored or stigmatised. For older people with dementia, the problem is even worse: they face the double jeopardy of being old and cognitively impaired. (Hoogeveen 2006, p.1)

Dr David Lee's innovative and extensive study introduced earlier gives us much to consider regarding older people's sexuality. Of 7000 women and men who were sent questionnaires, fewer than 3 per cent did not respond to direct questions about their sex lives and problems. The outcome of this exceptional study has revealed that not only are older men and women enjoying their sex lives, but that there are few places that they can turn to for support and information regarding their sexual challenges. Lee is vehement in his belief that health professionals themselves must become more open to discussing sexual health with older people and to act on their findings. He believes that these discussions should not be treated as irrelevancies.

It is also not uncommon that the reproductive and genitourinary health of older adults suddenly diminishes as a concern for those over 70 and especially those in communal living and persons living with dementia. No one who engages in sexual partnership is immune from sexually transmitted disease or HIV infection unless they have a long-term exclusive relationship. Who advises late-life partners about practising safe sex and the use of condoms in particular?

Disease and dysfunction of the reproductive and genitourinary systems of men and women may have a negative effect on healthy sexuality. How many of us know if mammograms, pelvic exams and prostate and rectal checks occur routinely in later life, especially for those women and men residing in care homes? These examinations and investigations can pose a challenge for many of us at the best of times. Yet a person living with dementia may find themselves exempt from these preventative investigations which could highlight conditions to be remedied when discovered early. Symptoms of such conditions can dramatically encroach on the ability to engage in and enjoy sex. Are age and diagnosis legitimate reasons to exclude men and women from these health screenings?

Points for Reflection

Without judgement, but with mindful awareness and acceptance, have a look at the statements and questions below to help guide your reflections.

» Notice your overall impression of this chapter – what does that feel like to you?

» Were there parts that might have made you feel uncomfortable, defensive, challenged? If so, what were they?

» Were there parts that were aligned with your own way of thinking, behaving, values or beliefs? If so, what were they?

» Were there any shocks or surprises? If so, what made them feel that way to you?

» Would you like to think differently about any of the issues that were discussed?

» What would you like to think/say/do differently?

» If you support staff in your professional role, how might you engage with them around these topics?

Chapter 2

In the Beginning... Biology

'I'll just DIE if I don't have sex RIGHT NOW!' We may have said or heard these words during our life time; we may have felt them to be true, or perhaps this is still in the future. As far as we know, an individual has not died for lack of sex exactly when they had wished to engage in it, but in a broader, whole species sense, there are implications for survival. This chapter will look at those elements of biology, our human needs that are 'hard wired' into our brains and behaviour, and discuss the implications that living with dementia has on biology and the brain.

We will look at what is happening in the brain regarding sex and the brain, and sex and dementia, to get an underlying sense of the basics we might want to know about.

We have learned many positive lessons in the ways of supporting men and women living with dementia through addressing their basic human needs as defined by 'biological imperatives'. They are the things that a person or a society needs in order for it to survive individually or as a group.

They are the need to eat, drink, eliminate, sleep and copulate – or have sex.

The so-called 'biological imperatives' of ontogeny and species survival have enormous influence on our sexual development and also our need and how we respond to that need if it exists. The need to eat, drink, eliminate, copulate and sleep form our 'must do' list. Although an individual might not die from lack of sex, the particular family legacy and contribution to the gene pool and species might. Our innate drive to eat, drink, sleep and eliminate are also within our learned control and attest to our socialisation and development if we are able to manage and defer gratification of these 'musts' to appropriate time and place. Eventually, biology will win and, in the face of extremis, our fierce instinct for survival will motivate our behaviour towards these ends. Our increasing 21st-century sophistication means that our psycho-social-emotional selves will also influence and shape those imperatives towards a higher ideal or the common good. The need and desire to copulate is even more heavily monitored. We also might live celibate lives either through circumstance or choice, totally, or in part and within an existing relationship for a time.

Not everyone wants to or chooses to engage in sexual activity. The majority of adults do. It is a normal part of our humanity and often joyous and desirable. The media and Freud would have us believe that it is our primary motivating force, and there is something wrong with us if it isn't. Our introduction into the world of being sexual begins in utero, when the developing foetus is female. At eight weeks, testosterone, the male hormone, is released and the foetus begins to take on male characteristics if destined by the genes to become male. As newborn infants we should have all we need within us to become fully functioning sexual beings following puberty when further hormones will charge up our sexual maturity. We are sexual individuals until our last breath. What we do with that sexuality in between is another part of the story.

How we become physically sexually functioning men and women or not (valuing men and women who are asexual) may include choices highly influenced by gender, expectations, politics, family values, faith, economics, culture. Choice may be taken out of our control by people and circumstances that do not respect the individual, age, gender, family, society or the law.

Our sexual expressions may be a kaleidoscope of more and less exciting, loving and satisfactory or traumatic sexual experiences over our lifetime.

We may engage with others or please only ourselves, or both, over the course of our sexual lives.

Interestingly, even the biological imperatives need reminders in the later stages of living with dementia when the areas of the brain controlling and triggering appetite, thirst, elimination and sleep are less reliable. The desire for sex may also diminish and not seem to be missed. That does not mean that touch and being held and hugged will not be an important addition to ensuring wellbeing. Indeed, we know that people can and do die from lack of caring touch. In our Western culture, we have learned, over millennia, to delay gratification and ensure that we have enough to eat and drink and get enough sleep. Some of us have had the ability to produce children, not only ensuring the survival of our own individual lineage and legacy, but contributing to the gene pool and the survival of the species.

Along the way we have also learned that sex is not only about reproduction but also about sexual pleasure, lust, romance, power, belonging, a rite of passage and earning money.

Nowadays it is possible to know the gender of the baby before it is born, and the gender shaping will begin once the word is out. Other babies have to wait until they are born, but for most there seems to be no escape from gender shaping, and the old nature-versus-nurture debate continues to be tested yet remains open to interpretation. We also know that for some males and females those gender designations may become oppressive and confining, and that the mismatch between genitalia and psychological and emotional felt gender identity may be at odds. Other men and women may be sexually equipped beings but feel no sexual desire at all and would wish to be known as asexual.

Preference for both sexes, the same sex or opposite sex exclusively or in combination are also rich distillations of our unique biology. However many variations on a theme we might describe, we are at risk of using heterosexual expression as the status quo. In actual fact, it is our brain, our neurology, which forms the baseline sexuality from which our creativity in sexual expression emerges as unique. The unique human embodies his or her sexuality in particular ways, resulting in the preferences we have within a vast array of possibilities and potentialities. Some of these emerge as sexual thoughts, feeling, behaviours. But they are only part of the whole person – our sexuality also influences our attitudes, emotions, spirituality, intellect, consumer choices. Please forgive the simplistic descriptions here – I acknowledge that there are numerous academic and detailed popular texts available. My intention is to draw attention to the layers of sexual possibilities men and women living with dementia may experience.

By the time we are born, we have all that we need to become sexually active and to procreate. Our sexual stimulation and pleasure centres begin even in utero and then as newborn babies. We know that male infants have erections, and that baby girls experience vaginal lubrication, especially during breast feeding. Orgasm can inadvertently or intentionally result at a very young age from rubbing or touching the genitals.

We cease being sexual creatures when we breathe our last. Note that being a sexual creature does not mean that sexual pleasure alone or with other(s) is a given. Our sexual history emerges as unique to each of us and is shaped by numerous experiences.

If we can see, then, that our desire and need for sex is 'hard wired', as with the need for food, drink, elimination and sleep, we can perhaps appreciate that those needs, thoughts and feelings are not usually easily switched off. It takes will and strength and determination to ignore the sex drive once it is aroused. But we can find other things to do in the moment if it's not appropriate to be sexual right away. I'm sure you can think of your own distractions without too much trouble. In my sexuality workshops, I always ask participants what we do when we can't have sex. The list is long, interesting and generally humorous. This is, as it happens, a very important exercise. If we know and can imagine what those alternatives are, then some of those can be offered when the opportunity for sex and orgasm is not immediately available for those living with later-stage dementia, especially if they are living in a care community or alone at home.

As you can imagine, this takes a great deal of brain power and a lot of that is surging in the front part of the brain, where the inhibiting mechanism resides, keeping us socially and culturally appropriate. The brain centres for memory (hippocampus) and emotion (limbic system and amygdala) and the production of hormones will all be hard at work, saying, 'Not now! Later!'

When brain function is affected by the processes of dementia, these complex messages may become confused or confusing, as felt need and actions are allowed their freedom, having sneaked under the radar of the ever-watchful inhibiting mechanism, resulting in what is termed 'disinhibition'. Alternatively, the ensuing confusion may result in a person shutting out and shutting down, and withdrawing as a means of staying safe and/or simplifying life. This may not be an altogether conscious act or a choice, but rather a default position learned previously in life. If it has worked well and served a purpose in the past, it will have been rehearsed and stored to be recalled at a later date. This recall will not last indefinitely as the ability of the brain (hippocampus primarily) to retrieve information diminishes over time.

The Brain, Dementia and Sex

When I think about how much information is too much and how much might be helpful, given these vast and complex areas of research and science, I hope that I have arrived at the correct balance. What I have chosen to include and what to omit is based on many of my training courses and from support groups for relatives and people living with dementia over many years and on two continents. I do apologise that I have left out *most* of it. Those of you who are particularly interested can explore to your heart's delight and never run out of fascinating information. Two of my favourite sources of information are the Alzheimer's Association *Inside the Brain: An Interactive Tour* (see website section in the References) and *Neuroscience for Dummies* (Amthor 2012).

What remains, I believe, are the essential things it might be helpful to know about our brains and dementia, especially what happens to our brains during sex and how these activities may be interrupted or become less available or less interesting as life changes us or dementia arrives. The more we stimulate certain pathways and activities, the more likely they are to be embedded in our memory store and repeated – especially if they are pleasurable. Sex is a big contender in the 'pleasure to be repeated' category. Certain behaviours (including sex) are more readily available as they are rehearsed and repeatedly stored. This is the opposite of the old adage 'if you don't use it, you lose it'. This may well be true, but I also like that other old adage that says that 'it's just like riding a bicycle: you climb back on and you remember how to do it'.

I think that sex is a bit like them both. It's getting the balance right that counts.

As we age, our sex lives change. A retired lesbian couple told me they were having the time of their lives with no alarm clocks in the morning or children to collect from school. Their daytime sex was fresh and fun and knocked the spots off golf or gardening, even though they also enjoyed those activities. In Western society, men and women in retirement communities, holiday clubs and on cruise ships are part of the group who have more leisure time and financial assets than ever before in history – and they are enjoying their sex lives very much, thank you. However, we might also expect changes in levels of fatigue, libido, erectile and lubrication problems, climax and arousal times, mobility, pain and the effects of medication. These changes can also occur across the adult lifespan in relation to a number of different scenarios. Dementia will at some point impose added difficulties in every area of life, including bodily functions and relating to others. The sexual, relational changes do not happen all at once or indeed to all people living with dementia, and they do not affect people in the same ways.

How will we support those elders who are currently living it up, when they develop dementia? Will their energy and enthusiasm and literal 'lust' for life just take a back seat?

As the Boy Scouts know only too well, preparation is everything. And prepare, we must, through developing our sensitivity, our knowledge and practical responses and dialogue. For today and tomorrow. It may be your future and mine.

The brain is the only organ that thinks about itself and how it works. It also thinks about how all the other parts of the body, mind and spirit work. The liver, under the control of the brain, only does liver functions. The muscles only do muscle functions, and the lungs only do lung functions. You get the idea. The brain does all of it *and* the brain functions. It does most of its work without our conscious awareness (thank goodness), and a great deal of it while we are asleep, including repairing itself during deep sleep phases called rapid eye movement (REM) sleep. We would get nothing done if we were aware of how much hydrochloric acid was dropping into our stomachs after lunch, or how many times our eyes have just blinked, or the number of skin cells dividing at this moment. You can see how tricky life could be. The brain is also the seat of the 'mind', thought, consciousness, personality, the soul. What an astounding thing it is. It is gratifying to know that even when faced with dementia, the brain can and will adapt and develop to changes within and outside itself.

So, the brain is the biggest sex organ and controls all aspects of our chemical, hormonal, psychological, emotional, spiritual and physical selves. From the interaction between the stimulation of our senses and thoughts all the way through to sexual behaviour and climax, our sexual responses might resemble the finely crafted symphony of many parts being brought together to achieve the whole performance under the leadership of the conductor (the brain). The brain needs to be fairly functional, although not totally perfect in order for us to engage with our sexual selves and perhaps others. When we develop dementia, our sexual selves and behaviour also become part of the shifting inner–outer world that may become less familiar over time. We may retain our responses and desires but lose recognition of who was the object of our affection previously, responding more to physical arousal and being less controlled by our former inhibitory responses. Some deep-seated memories of our sexual selves may remain, still fully formed, or fragmented and possibly misaligned to the current place, time or partner. Our sexual responses and desires may abandon us in part or completely. The role our brain has in this process is key to our understanding and supporting persons with dementia.

Brain Basics

Weighing in at 2.5kg and feeling and looking like a bowl of porridge left over from yesterday, the brain is the exquisite and marvellous source of it all, our Commander in Chief. But if it's not happening in the headroom, it's not happening in the bedroom.

The powerhouse that is our brain, our control centre, the 'mother board', is a fascinating and highly complex combination of billions of electro-chemical impulses and interactions at any given moment in time.

Click your fingers. In that second, 1000 neuronal impulses or nerve cell interactions took place. The brain is made up of the cortex, or the mass of tissue that is 70 per cent water – the rest is nerve tissue, blood supply, oxygen and nutrients. Around 100 billion neurons or specialised nerve cells create an interactive web-like structure of connections within a complicated circuit of electro-chemical impulses which send and receive information from the five senses to the muscles and organs and back again. Many brain cells or neurons die daily, and we consistently lose neurons from the time we are born. This is normal and doesn't affect our ability to learn and retain new information.

Neurotransmitters or chemical messengers transfer information from one nerve cell or neuron to another at amazing speed, communicating important information which becomes thought, sensation, action all over the body and the brain. Other chemicals, called hormones, play a huge part in the regulation of the brain's millions of functions, and we are most familiar with those involved in puberty and pregnancy, such as oestrogen, progesterone and testosterone.

Also involved in sex are the brain's feel-good chemicals, or endorphins, which have multiple functions. Involved with our sex lives is a hefty cocktail of interactions and processes. You may recognise dopamine, the pleasure hormone which tells us we want 'more of the same please'; serotonin, the happy and relaxed hormone (under threat during depression); and oxytocin, the 'cuddle chemical', which is released not only to enhance mother-and-infant bonding but also during orgasm and sensual touch. Research suggests that it may be one of the reasons women tend to fall in love with their sexual partners and why we might be serially attracted to partners who aren't good for us once we leave the bedroom. It does, however, help release empathy in men, too, and the opportunity for bonding with their baby. It's also responsible for men falling asleep immediately after sex.

Testosterone, the male hormone involved with lots of other things as well as sex, keeps men wanting more sex but not necessarily cuddles. It is worth noting that it is also responsible for erections that have no connection with the man wanting to have sex. It's just how it is wired into the body (Brizendine 2010). This may have implications for how we support men living with dementia who may have forgotten that erections can occur unbidden and unannounced, and who may be miscued into believing that sexual behaviour is required to keep up with the messages the penis is sending. Frank and open discussion about this possibility and its origins can alleviate anxiety and embarrassment on the part of the man in question. The men who attend the dementia café, the golf club, the day centre or who become residents in the care home may experience these events. Without this foreknowledge, misunderstandings and incorrect assumptions can be made, resulting in embarrassment, confusion and enhanced vulnerability. It can lead to stereotyping and labelling of what is normal and unpredictable behaviour. The man living with dementia, in a later stage of dementia, may be less able to understand what is happening and may respond to the change as a trigger for sexual behaviour. The ability to support him at this time will be key to maintaining his dignity, self-esteem and safety, and that of others. This will require a conversation with the man in question as a part of getting to know him and creating a sexual profile. We know that there are likely to be changes to sexual thoughts, feelings and behaviour from whatever is the 'normal' or 'usual' for the individual concerned. It will be helpful to know that there may be changes in the area of sexuality and intimacy as well as in other aspects of living with dementia. We would be unlikely to withhold information that we knew could be useful and helpful to a person, their partner and/or carers about how living with dementia affects other aspects of activities of daily living.

Why would we choose to ignore sex, when so many adults consider it to be one of their activities of daily living too? Once we have our training behind us and have worked on our own willingness and abilities to have conversations about sex and sexuality or intimacy, we will find it becomes easier and just a part of the conversation about how living with dementia can change how and when we do things, where and with whom.

Surely this is also part of our duty of care to be as inclusive and comprehensive as we can be and not discriminate about the information we share. One of the areas or lobes of the brain particularly involved in sex is the fronto-temporal area, and the frontal lobe specifically. If we develop a form of fronto-temporal (the front and side of the brain) dementia, or Pick's disease specifically, initial changes taking place in the area at the front of the brain will create disinhibition.

An experience of 'disinhibition' is not uncommon in many forms of dementia. It can also be the result of trauma or tumour in this location and so neurological investigations must be undertaken to rule out these other causes, rather than assume that the disinhibition is caused by a frontal lobe dementia.

This will not be an alien experience to some of us who have had a delirium associated with an illness or a high temperature, or even a dental anaesthetic. Too much alcohol or recreational drugs designed to lower our inhibitions can give rise to a disinhibited state from which one usually recovers; this can also affect women in the throes of childbirth. Some types of mental health problems also include disinhibition as part of their experience. Thoughts, feelings and fantasies, including those of a sexual nature, were once safely tucked away and kept private by the 'inhibiting mechanism'. This keeps us socially and culturally safe and appropriate. Imagine for a moment that your innermost private sexual thoughts, feelings and fantasies, usually well protected by the inhibiting mechanism of your brain, are now, as a result of dementia, available for all to hear and see. This may also include your opinions about the appearance of others and your feelings towards them! Frontal lobe dementia syndromes also tend to present in younger people, sometimes beginning in the late 40s. Arriving as it does in mid-life, diagnosis is a long process of elimination, and the main features at the beginning are less likely to include memory loss and confusion or difficulty with language, the usual signposts to a dementia. Often a diagnosis of 'mid-life crisis' seems to fit.

Barbara tearfully described 'losing' her husband Bill to Pick's disease, beginning when he was 56. It took seven years to diagnose. During this time, the main features of the condition were dramatic personality changes, aggression, sexual disinhibition and promiscuity, drinking, going to night clubs and arguing at work. His memory and ability to use language were fairly intact for a long time. He also argued with Barbara as she tried to point out the problems in their marriage and at his work, as she tried to understand this behaviour and failed.

> Women from his office would ring me up and tell me to talk to my husband about his wandering hands or sexual invitations or they would report him. He had been well liked, a good boss – and this was a shock to everyone.
>
> Most of all me. Sometimes he would stay out all night. Our sex life changed dramatically to the point where I prayed he wouldn't come near me, and I would often stay out at neighbours' or friends', until I thought he would fall asleep on the sofa. Then I would creep into the spare room. He said awful, sick and demeaning things to me. He was drinking a lot, and that didn't help the arguments. I couldn't stand it anymore and went to talk to the GP when

Bill was sacked from his job. Bill refused to go to the GP: I had a problem, he didn't. It was all my fault and he told everyone what a terrible woman I was – and worse. Things about our private life.

I had to find work. He then hit me during one of our arguments, and I'd had enough. I went to stay with my sister who is a social worker and who knew Bill well.

He couldn't care for himself or the flat, and finally we were able to get social services in to assess him. He was malnourished, dehydrated and had obviously not been showering or washing his clothes or bedding or taking out the trash or clearing old food out. The flat was an environmental hazard, and his physical and mental health was obviously at risk. He was hospitalised. He is now in a care home and does not know me when I go to visit. I am devastated. We were so looking forward to our retirement. He was a lovely man.

From this stark and upsetting story, we can begin to appreciate how important it is to understand the different forms that dementia can take and during which time of life. We are only beginning to see dementia-specific education and training in medical and nursing schools, and in psychology and allied health professionals' courses of study. As certain forms of dementia involve the sexual aspects of behaviour and relating earlier than other types, it would have been so important for Barbara and Bill to have had access to health professionals who were knowledgeable and skilled.

This scenario underscores the importance of early and accurate diagnosis, the absence of which can multiply the challenges to be faced.

I would like to point out that this is just one person's experience of Pick's disease and not all will follow this exact pattern. The challenge presents itself in our understanding of different types of dementia. It provides the necessary evidence that not all forms of dementia are the same, and therefore we need to understand the finer points of each type in order to provide the most appropriate interventions, services and support. This is especially true of young-onset dementia, when Bill's behaviour might be described as a mid-life crisis or a mental health issue rather than developing dementia. Barbara was asked to use her experiences to help others by her public speaking engagements and involvement in the Pick's Society (now known as Rare Dementia Support). She knew that, finally, Bill was receiving the care he needed, and she was happy to leave things like that to professionals.

It is not unusual in any form of dementia for a person to think that others are causing or creating the problem, and that they are well and capable, and refuse to go to the GP. And, indeed, when they eventually do, they are often able to maintain a high degree of socially appropriate behaviour that puts a diagnosis of dementia in question and the mental state of the person who brought them in doubt. This is not done in any way to be argumentative or obstinate. It is a normal way of the brain to try to make sense of Self when none of it adds up to being sensible at all.

Let's look more closely at some of the brain function and behaviour that will affect sex and living with dementia.

The limbic system, which includes the amygdala, hippocampus and limbic lobe folded into the centre of the cortex – described as 'our most primitive' brain system – is the focal point of our emotional selves, steering us away from painful events and directing us towards the pleasurable ones, including sex.

A fascinating report in *Dementia Today* (2013), an American online resource, pools years of research and highlights the good news that researchers have realised that the brain is highly 'plastic' or flexible and adaptable. Where we once thought that neurons (nerve cells in the brain) were not able to be replaced or repaired, we now know that an enriched environment of cortical (brain) stimulation, exercise and healthy diet and lifestyle can create new neurons (neurogenesis) and strengthen or create new connections between existing neurons. Good communication between neurons can improve learning and memory. Learning new information and having to adapt to new situations can have this strengthening and renewing effect on brain cells. Brain training and specific tasks designed to increase opportunities for new learning have been shown to be beneficial in keeping the hippocampus healthy. The hippocampus is affected considerably when living with dementia as it is one of the most important primitive areas of the brain associated with memory formation, storage and retrieval – all functions that become diminished with the onset and progression of dementia, especially of the Alzheimer's type.

A healthy hippocampus, and, more generally, a healthy brain, we are told, can also reduce plaques formed of beta-amyloid protein that become toxic in brains of people with Alzheimer's disease. It can increase the production of proteins and blood vessels that can support growth and survival of healthy nerve cells.

The superb craftsmanship of the brain and the interactions that take place for all of our thoughts, feelings and behaviours, as well as the complex functioning of our bodies, cannot be overstated or overrated. I know this only too well from a personal experience several years ago. I would like to share some of it here as I feel it is particularly relevant and may even be helpful to some. A number of years ago I sustained a minor head injury. I hit my head on the corner of a concrete staircase in a car park. I didn't fall over, and I wasn't concussed or unconscious. However, what ensued was very worrying and uncomfortable and told me a lot about my brain, the organ I had taken so completely for granted in myself, but perhaps less so in other people.

I later joked that this was God's way of keeping my work authentic.

During my medical investigations, I made the acquaintance of a wonderful neurologist who was so patient and empathic and informative. Apparently, minor head injuries are hugely under-reported but can cause real problems for several months or years, even though nothing shows up on a scan. So, apart from dizziness, headache, confusion, difficulty finding words, memory problems, mood swings, problems sleeping and depression, I was thrown into early menopause at 48 and had some challenges with sex – not feeling much like it for one thing, and then a much longer time to get in the mood and to reach climax. This lasted for around six months, but the menopause went on into full production, with all that entails.

Although recovery was complete, this experience gave me an opportunity to really become aware of my own brain function and how troubling it was when I had a knock on the head that did not allow me to behave or function as I would normally. I also thought about how it might feel to a person with dementia when they may have been experiencing changes for up to five years before seeking a diagnosis. I thought about the numerous MRI scans and other computer imaging I have seen where the loss of brain tissue was dramatic and quite undeniable. I thought about the changes to the sex lives of all of those people I had worked with over the years. Some chose to tell me about their experiences; others did not. That doesn't mean that changes were not taking place and possibly wreaking havoc with self-confidence, performance, relationships and intimacy. But I would not have known if they were in trouble.

I am not advocating that we ask everyone with dementia about their sex life, but not even considering it or realising that it will be affected by dementia is a real oversight on our part. Sometimes simply making a decision to be open and become informed ourselves can influence the conversations we have about relationships, how intimacy with friends, family and partners changes over time. That may open the door to a more in-depth conversation about sex.

I believe that our awareness and knowledge of what might happen in the brain or between the sheets, so to speak, is *essential*, and usually invisible, sometimes even to ourselves and our sexual partners. We can only hope to enhance our empathy and commitment to working with and relating to people from a person-centred approach, resulting in a more rounded and grounded view of the sexuality of others and of ourselves.

So far we have had an opportunity to explore some of the brain basics as they are affected by dementia, and how that may in turn affect our sexual thoughts, feelings and behaviours. In terms of the brain and consciousness and integrated functioning, there is a very complicated school of thought that embraces philosophy and psychology called embodied cognition. The basic premise is that the body and brain are integrated within the lived environment and that we separate them at our peril.

What if we considered that, without our body, our abilities to think, dream, communicate and function would cease to exist. Our body and brain are one – are who we are. Our brain and our cognition exist within the physical body that houses and nourishes the brain and transports it throughout our lives, events and relationships. Embodied.

We are in error if we place all primacy within the brain. To be human means to walk through the world intact with the full orchestration of body, brain and spirit. Holistic approaches reflect this integration. Within the world of living with dementia, there is often a focus that the brain is the only repository of knowledge and memory. This is easy to appreciate, as the brain is the organ affected by conditions causing dementia that result in the challenges to daily living, relationships and personhood. Of course, the brain will ultimately process incoming and outgoing information and also the information we carry around within us, the knowledge and the internal conversations that remain within. All of those thoughts and feelings you are having right now, as well as what you are reading in this sentence. All of the learning we have stored over the years, that may or may not be shared or used. There is an internal world of events that only you will know. There is also the life history narrative that each of us carries and builds on throughout our lives.

To separate the brain from the body will result in only a partial story. It may result in some independent functioning, but will diminish the whole. Integration. The heart of the matter is the heart. Without its life-giving pumping of blood throughout the body and the brain, nothing will happen. The vital role of blood pressure to ensure that the heart's actions move the blood supply along is in itself a highly complex, interactive process. Without the brain's ability to inform the heart and circulatory system how to function, it would be deprived of its blood supply and die. But what of the lungs, breathing oxygen into the body to be carried to the brain by the blood stream, and the kidneys which purify the blood and urine of harmful toxins and waste? These vital and essential bodily functions cannot happen without the control system of the brain, and it and its millions of component parts will die without it.

What are the eye and brain doing to translate these black marks on a piece of paper or a screen (what *is* paper, a screen, and how do you know?) into something you understand? How many thoughts and feelings spin off each word? You can feel your body as it fits inside what you may be wearing, how it feels in the chair or on the bus as you are reading. You also hold the information of when to get off the bus, or get up from the chair, where you are going next and what you will be doing in millions of moments, hours, days, weeks and months ahead. Did you take the chicken out of the freezer for dinner? You smile at the memory of your lover's kiss, your sunrise walk with the dog and how that pulled muscle feels.

And you are reading, scratching your head, lifting your coffee cup and drinking, or moving over on the seat to let another passenger sit beside you on the bus, aware of his wet raincoat on your arm and umbrella dripping on your foot. The role of the mind and spirit, or soul, in this extraordinary orchestration of solo parts is magnificent.

When dis-embodied, when we separate the 'brain function' from the whole person living with dementia, we are in danger of diminishing the person, anticipating disability and challenge where none may exist. If this is the case, we can appreciate how that anticipation shapes our own and others' expectations, often reducing brain and behaviour to the lowest common denominator. We may believe (erroneously) that knowledge and understanding of brain function and its resulting behaviour or thinking are the whole story.

I am continually surprised and awestruck by experiences of persons living with dementia which demonstrate and confirm that we need to think and act in more integrated terms and alter our expectations accordingly.

The late and marvellous neurological pioneer and poet Oliver Sacks encourages us to expect the unexpected. If we expect integration rather than dis-integration, residual strength instead of apparent loss, that expectation can fill in the gaps to create a whole experience. Reliance only on more obvious changes in neurological functioning serves to dis-integrate and to diminish our expectations.

Early in the 1980s, when I was first working with people with dementia in the USA, I had a remarkable experience which changed for ever my expectations of the abilities of persons living with dementia to process information, to respond out of the blue and to encourage me to expect the unexpected.

Mike's wife, Beth, came to the care home every day to visit him. We would all have coffee and home-made goodies and talk to Mike and include him in our chat. To all intents and purposes, Mike appeared to be asleep in his recliner chair. Occasionally, when Beth kissed him, he would open his eyes wide and smile at her and call her 'darling'. Those were precious moments. One morning, Beth was telling us both that she was packing to go to Florida for a couple of weeks with their daughter, to get away from the New England winter. To our amazement, Mike sat bolt upright in his chair and looked Beth right in the eyes. 'Have a wonderful time in Florida, darling,' he said and then reclined again with his eyes closed.

> You can imagine our delight and surprise – especially Beth's. That was to be the last time Mike ever spoke to Beth or seemed to recognise her verbally. Precious moments indeed, built on the expectation that Mike was listening. Just because he wasn't letting us know he was did not alter the fact that Beth and I believed that, somewhere in there, Mike was processing what was happening.

Muscle memory, emotional memory, sensory memory can stimulate connections through the whole body, mind and spirit in ways that direct cognitive stimulation alone may not manage. Being part of nature and the immediate world outside of the body allows for interactions and responses that can stimulate and calm the brain and many of its functions, including the emotions which may be less available or more available in people living with dementia.

You may recall the memories of the philosopher Marcel Proust as he savours the freshly baked French cakes called Madeleines and how his memory of these cakes is often cited to make a point about sensory memory, olfactory (sense of smell) specifically, as I am doing now. That one sensory memory then embraces sight and touch and taste and hearing. But where does it originate? In the same vein, think about the smell of your favourite thing baking in the oven... Is it your grandmother's apple pie or your mother's meatloaf? The smell of a particular aftershave will take me immediately on a trip down memory lane to teenage years, a first boyfriend and where we went dancing with our friends in Brighton.

Only we humans are consciously aware of ourselves as we live these lives in each moment. We ask these questions and attempt to make sense of our lives: what is life and how does it occur, in relation to others and the world? The mind – our thought processes, emotions, spirituality, imagination and dreams – is a daunting, awesome and marvellous and perhaps terrifying thing. Especially so when our ability to be in control of some of it unravels.

Yet together, in our relationships as comrades-in-arms, we can embark on new journeys of discovery, become pioneers of our own interiority. Most fascinating is the inter-relationship between neurobiology and personhood and how, in spite of what we should expect based on neuroscience alone, the human spirit, sheer determination and adaptation keep us in thrall. No less fascinating is this infinite mystery of our human sexuality and how it is affected, diminished or enhanced as the brain, body and spirit adapt to living with dementia, leaving us in a state of wonder and gratitude that things are not always as they seem.

Points for Reflection

Without judgement, but with mindful awareness and acceptance, have a look at the statements and questions below to help guide your reflections.

> » Notice your overall impression of this chapter – what does that feel like to you?

> » Did your understanding of the 'biological imperatives' improve or stay the same?

> » How does brain and behaviour enhance your present understanding of what can happen when affected by living with dementia?

> » Are there aspects of a person's behaviour that you see differently now?

» How has this chapter informed your thinking about, and responding to, sex and the person living with dementia?

» What would you like to think/say/do differently?

» If you support staff in your professional role, how might you engage with them around these topics?

3

Responding to the Need for Sensuality, Sexuality and Intimacy

I may be a sensual person in my appreciation and desire for my senses to be stimulated – by Egyptian cotton sheets, candlelight and fresh flowers wherever possible, music, delicious things to eat and drink presented artistically, massage, bubble baths with candles and wine, the touch of a newborn's cheek against my own, a sunrise, a thunderstorm, the love of my pets and snuggling with them, the scent of aftershave, a log fire.

Stop reading for a minute and write down what creates sensuality in your life. If you have a partner, write each other's lists. Share them and talk about how you already do or could do more to enhance each other's sensual wellbeing, which may lead to sex, but doesn't have to.

Many care homes are wonderfully imaginative in their supply of the sensual, from beauty treats to Snoezelen rooms (based on the Dutch concept from the 1970s of multisensory stimulation for persons with intellectual disabilities) to a beach hut created in a storage room with sounds of waves and seagulls, sand, seaweed and stones, deck chairs and an ice-cream cart, or an indoor 'pub' complete with dart board, bar snacks and snooker table.

Sensuality can enhance our feelings of wellbeing and/or can become a precursor to sexual activity. It is no coincidence that dating often includes multiple sensual experiences, and I am sure you can add many more.

I can be a sensual, sexual person and be celibate.

I can be a sensual and sexually active person.

I can be a sensual person and asexual.

I can be living with dementia and still be any of the above.

Our senses are there being stimulated randomly, or with intention, with or without awareness, with or without sex.

Positive sensual experiences can result in feelings of pleasure and wellbeing.

As described earlier, for some, the challenge of speaking to their elders about sex and intimacy in our professional role seems intrusive, embarrassing and frankly uncomfortable. However, it is essential that we separate ourselves from the voice inside that says, 'I wouldn't like that to happen to my mum,' or 'Dad doesn't think like that – he's pretty well past it now.'

Speaking to someone younger than yourself about living with dementia and the effect this is having on their sex life is not an easy conversation either. However, if we are to be truly person-centred and holistic in our approach, we must at least be thinking about sexuality and our client group, if not actually having the conversations, and we must be receiving training, supervision and training others in turn.

Georgina was a drama teacher in the local high school. Brett was a lawyer specialising in company law. They had two daughters age six and nine. They had a lovely home, a dog and a busy life with active children, extended family and friends. Georgina was diagnosed with early-onset dementia just after her 40th birthday. She and her husband had been thinking about trying for a baby before menopause. She was younger than me by 15 years when I heard about her situation. I was really challenged by my own experiences of people living with dementia and my expectations of who might be affected. Dementia and its impact on sex for a woman of child-bearing age had not yet featured in my reality; although I had heard that the youngest person to be diagnosed with Alzheimer's disease was 28, it was still relatively theoretical to me. This was much closer to home and it made a huge impact on me.

At the time I heard their story, Georgina and Brett had decided not to make any major decisions until they could take in the full implications for Georgina herself, for them as a couple and them all as a family. They hoped to start family counselling soon, and Georgina had already begun individual counselling and was working with her school and her union to see what her options were. She was looking into disability rights. It was a complete shock to this woman who reportedly said, 'This is not meant to be happening to me. I eat well, exercise, I never smoked and I hardly ever drink. How can this s**t beat me to the menopause!' Her mother, grandmother, and an aunt (her mother's older sister) and her daughter (Georgina's cousin) had previously been diagnosed with young-onset dementia. Her grandmother had died; her mother was in a care home. She didn't know about her aunt and her cousin; they were not close as they had lived in Australia since Georgina was a baby and were only in contact at the holidays. It is not unusual in this type of familial scenario that some members choose to ignore the probabilities of genetic inheritance and refuse any testing or counselling that is offered. Georgina also did not want to know what might happen to her young daughters.

When situations arise that truly surprise or shock us, professional supervision is the best place to go where we can process our feelings, recognise what we may have done well and imagine what we might have done better. We can reflect on our learning, what we could do the next time in a similar situation and find ways to help us to move forward. Our lives may be touched by many and we may not always know what happens to clients or patients. We will always wonder how their lives progressed. We remember them with kindness and hope that they find the care and support they need and deserve wherever they are, and we cheer them on.

We know more about the lives and deaths of those we support in residential and nursing care environments, and there are many occasions of fun, celebration, good living and the best in end-of-life care. Supporting hundreds of care home managers throughout the UK in a leadership development programme called My Home Life based at City University of London is an inspiration and joy to me. I hear of excellent and innovative care and relationships with people living with dementia and their families. In a culture that derides the care home sector and fears dying with dementia, I am in awe of what good living and gracious dying can be achieved with skill, compassion, good person-centred care and the nurturing of relationships with residents, relatives and staff towards wellbeing.

It is exactly because we are not partners or family or grown-up children that we can take that necessary step back to assess the rights and needs of the adult before us. This is maybe a step too far for family and not always easy to manage on their own. If, for some reason, training around sexuality has not reached all of your staff, find the person within your organisation who is interested, willing and skilled in this area. It doesn't have to be the manager, the GP or assumed senior person in charge. This approach, of course, needs to be respectful of all involved, knowledgeable and caring, but at the same time holding out for the rights and needs of the identified adult in our care. The person for whom we have a duty of care also has the right to privacy within our service or living facility. Balancing the needs and concerns of anxious and upset relatives or children or teenage children and family members who are not next of kin requires sensitivity and consideration. Undoubtedly, not everyone will be happy with their family members' decisions and behaviour or our upholding of them when they are safe and legal.

If we purport to work in holistic and person-centred ways, then the whole of the human being must be included in our care assessment and provision, and in the writing of care and service plans. We also know that we deny the existence of sex and sensuality at our peril. We may, however, discover that sex itself is not hugely important, but having private time to snuggle and nap with a partner is essential to wellbeing. For others, the opportunity to use a vibrator or watch an adult film in privacy may be important. All are valid affirmations of any or all aspects of 'identity, comfort, inclusion, attachment, occupation and love', as described by Tom Kitwood (1997, p.82).

When we hear of behaviour described as challenging and distressing, I often wonder how much of the frustration, agitation, anger, depression and withdrawal are direct responses to the loss of sexual engagement in one's life. Adult humans in general can respond to lack of sexual gratification in the same ways. Why wouldn't we imagine the same could be true for adults living with dementia or other disability? Even without the possibility of sex and orgasm, our sensual selves are still available for exploration and celebration. Finding out who the person is and what soothes and comforts them in times of stress and anxiety, we can build a repertoire of good things to suggest or offer when times get tough.

These options are varied and highly individual, and often can be simple and free. Journal articles abound on the use of sensual stimulation to restore wellbeing.

Relationships with Family, Lovers and Staff

Love makes the world go round, we are told, and so does flirting. Spend time with our European elders for confirmation. Some of the most relaxed, supportive and comfortable environments I have visited have been places where non-offensive flirting and sexual banter takes place. This behaviour is a continuation of healthy human social interactions, which may or may not lead to sex. It allows men and women to feel vibrant, potent, attractive and valued. When people use humour, respect and common sense, it is an enjoyable experience for many men and women living with dementia. With the wellbeing of the individuals in mind, we can learn a great deal from those we support, their previous lives and current losses and longings, their capacity to survive and to empathise with and support one another.

Partners and relatives will be helped greatly by having conversations and relationships with empathic, skilled professionals, which highlight cognitive changes and needs of the person for sex, sensuality and intimacy, non-sexual touch, holding and cuddling. Supporting families, partners and friends with respect, information, knowledge, compassion and care can go a long way towards meeting the complex needs of persons living with dementia and enhancing their quality of life.

According to Kitwood, people who experience increased socialisation and affection are enjoying greater wellbeing.

Conversations with relatives and partners and persons living with dementia need to address sexuality, needs, fears and how to sustain their sexual selves before a move to an assisted living facility, residential or nursing care takes place. It is indeed a challenge to imagine that your life partner may find someone else to attach themselves to and may indeed wish to have sex with them instead of you. How would it feel to have a new sexual partner while still loving and caring for your partner with advanced dementia who is living at the nursing home now?

Environment and Sex

My experience of supporting staff in various care environments around sex and those they support is that those staff are often considerate, caring, skilled and open.

Where fear and anxiety exist as a result of poor or absent staff training, this is often projected on to the person living with dementia and their partner or relatives. Knowing your staff and their background and values will be an important aspect of the education, self-awareness and training that is offered, and allow the opportunity for supervision to offer one-to-one support to a staff member who may be struggling.

Many women and men with dementia are living at home for longer into the course of their dementia than ever before. Our attitudes, approaches and service provision need to embrace all types of living and supportive environments. If and when they move to an assisted living scheme or residential care facility, they are likely to be more frail and have more complex needs requiring care and skill.

Not all persons will live in a care home or nursing home, and we may never hear of any sexual issues or concerns while men and women are able to live without the input of health and social care with their privacy intact. Sex and relationships and/or opportunities for sex usually only come to our attention when there are problems or concerns associated with them.

As conditions progress, attending a day centre, lunch club, dementia café or living communally can create the stimulus of there being potential partners available, while the person does not remember that they are in a marriage or partnership already. It may also mean that changes in memory lead a person to mistake a fellow resident or group member for their partner, husband or wife, or one they knew long in the past.

How those in the supportive environment prepare for and respond to these events will be crucial to the wellbeing and safety of all concerned. Enlightened environments will have trained staff in place and have had discussions with partners and family ahead of the person's arrival at the new environment. There will be private places and spaces for people to be together or on their own.

Domiciliary care workers and extra support staff may arrive at the home of a person or persons who may still enjoy an active sex life. Being alone in someone's home can create misunderstanding and anxiety on both sides. The care worker's experience and training can create a positive environment with respect for the sexuality of the individual adult with rights and the right to privacy in their own home. As mentioned previously, with all of the clients we support, negative experiences are not as frequent as might be imagined, and a well-trained and sensitive home carer can listen and signpost a client to professional support. Managers and supervisors must also find the means to ensure appropriate and frequent training and supervision, and ensure the safety of their staff as well as those people with dementia using the service.

Misunderstanding and Miscuing

The excellent document *The Last Taboo* (2011) sensitively and intelligently describes issues of a sexual nature for those living with dementia in care homes. It provides helpful and practical guidance for partners and families and creates a step-by-step person-centred approach to situations we might find challenging.

Its author, Sally-Marie Bamford, tells us that:

Care home residents often have complex care needs and trying to understand and respond to the more intimate and sexual aspects of a resident's personality and relationship can be challenging, both in terms of existing relationships and when relationships develop and there can be no hard and fast rules as each situation and resident is unique. (Bamford 2011, p.4)

Men and women may misunderstand their roles and relationships towards one another as fellow residents or members of a day centre group and imagine sexual partners where there are none. They may have lost a sense of where they fit into one another's circles of relationship within family and friendship groups. I remember Emily pointing at David, the husband of a woman who attended the day centre with her.

E: Did I have one of 'em? (*Pointing at David as he stood beside Kathy, his wife.*)

D: Did you have one of what, Emily? A green sweater? A pair of glasses?

E: (*Waving her hands about in an agitated way and still pointing.*) One of them, the man thing.

D: Oh, do you mean a husband, Emily?

E: Yeah, one of 'em. Have I got one? Is he mine? (*Pointing again at David.*)

D: Yes, you have a husband, Emily. His name is Fred. (*Emily is listening intently, not quite believing me.*) He will be here to collect you soon to take you home where you live with him.

E: Oh. Does he have a green sweater?

D: I don't know, Emily. Maybe he does.

Fred arrives and greets Emily with a kiss (not wearing a green sweater).

F: Hello, old girl, have you behaved yourself today?

E: Ooh, get off, what you doing, kissing me?

D: Emily that's your husband, Fred.

E: (*Guffaws out loud.*) Oh Lord, that ain't him. What would I be doin' with a bald, fat, toothless old git like him?

D: How do you remember Fred, then?

E: Bloody marvellous 'e was. Love at first sight.

F: It was the same for me, doll. Never looked back or at another woman in 58 years.

E: Never. Is that you, then?

F: Yep, it's me. A bit different now. Five kids and eight grandkids, four great-grands to prove it.

E: Never! Not with me you didn't!

D: Are you two going home together today?

E: I don't know 'im. I can't go with someone I don't know, can I?

This scenario happened at the end of every day at the centre. It required two cups of tea, several biscuits and photographs of the family in Emily's life story book. In it there were then and now photos of Fred side by side, their wedding photograph and one taken the previous Christmas with their extended family. Emily didn't always know who she was in these and never who everyone else was without being told. After they had shared this together, something triggered Emily's memory and it felt safe to leave with Fred.

Every day Emily would look for 'David' in the green sweater (when he didn't wear it, that was even more distressing). She thought that he was her husband.

Given the rigours of childbirth, I cannot imagine that a mother would not remember that she had given birth to *five* babies. It is not unusual for a woman living with dementia not to remember that.

When we become less inhibited, women can become the seductresses they may always have believed themselves to be, but were not allowed to be for all sorts of reasons. Men in care homes and community environments are most often those who are thought to initiate sexual and intimate relationships. Although they do, women do also. I do not know the numbers for comparison's sake. In my experience, it is not uncommon, and it is also not uncommon for the male in the scenario to be 'blamed' for the sexual overtures or actual behaviour. This behaviour, although it may seem shocking to others, especially family, may be a very important milestone for this woman. We must be aware of the potential for harm to the vulnerable and also to the initiator of the relationship if the woman is stopped from following her heart and desire. Women and men who have lived their lives identified as heterosexual may begin to form same-sex relationships and, unbeknown to us, have been cued or miscued into thinking about someone from their past with whom they had, or wished that they had, a sexual relationship.

The context in which behaviour occurs, rather than the behaviour itself, is what usually deems it 'inappropriate'. The person engaged in the behaviour rarely recognises that it is inappropriate and, given their former selves, would no doubt be embarrassed and mortified that what is so private has been made so public and may cause concern, harm and embarrassment to someone else.

In community living environments, we also may give the wrong information and impression if we insist that 'this is your home now'. Most of us have very specific ideas of what we can do in the privacy of our own homes. Although we would not argue that we hope residents feel 'at home', 'homey' or 'like home', and that they are comfortable and relaxed and feel able to be themselves, we need to take care that we do not add to a confused idea about this place literally being 'my home'. There are many things that are so obviously not like your own home, including lots of strangers living together, lots of other strangers telling you what to do, and even more strangers monitoring and regulating 'your home'. How you sleep and with whom, what you wear or do in bed or on the sofa in front of the TV, or whether you wear your indoor dress and earrings instead of your outdoor trousers and shirt are just a few examples. Whenever I hear of a person living with dementia in a care home described as 'rummaging' in other people's wardrobes and drawers, I wonder whether one of these women or men might be looking for the kind of clothing they are used to wearing in their own home. What would it be like for the trans person who is not out, but is now living in your care home, and their family has brought them what they believe to be the appropriate clothing?

Living with dementia in a community environment that is clearly not home, but supposed to be home, can add to and create confusion about behaviour not to be shared in public, and sometimes not even in private. How can this be 'home'?

The most frequent occurrences of unsought sexual attention are people grabbing or fondling staff's breasts, genitals or buttocks, inviting them to engage in sex acts with them, or making sexually suggestive or lewd comments. Our training needs to provide us with the opportunities to see these situations for what they most probably are: a series of misunderstandings and miscuing. This means that a cue or a prompt is delivered by a staff member or fellow resident, which before the onset of dementia would have indicated sexual harassment or someone getting too frisky and inappropriate at a party or club. The responses and reactions we might have to the latter would not be helpful or legal in the care setting. And yet sometimes the same response or reaction is elicited when the person who instigated the behaviour may not have capacity to know what he or she is saying or doing. No one should have to go to work and be sexually harassed, denigrated, attacked or made vulnerable. With the best training in place, we will have a better understanding of what misunderstandings and miscuing may have originated and what we can do to best support the individual and also keep ourselves safe. We need to know how to communicate effectively, and know how to take care of ourselves and the person we are supporting, and those peers in their community.

In many situations, the person with dementia is alone with someone, being undressed, is naked or being given personal care or a back rub or massage. In their mind and body, the last time they were naked, with another person touching them or massaging them, touching their genitals, buttocks or breasts, more intimacy and sex may well have followed. The need for closeness of an intimate and sexual nature can be easily misunderstood and misinterpreted in intimate situations such as personal care or skin massage or helping someone to use the toilet.

Being clear and focused in our role as well as being warm and kind is a very difficult art to master. But master it, we do. It is being done well and creatively in many care homes and community environments across the country. Many residents in care facilities enjoy hugging, being touched, holding hands with staff, other residents and visiting family and friends. This need and desire to touch and be touched in non-sexual and sexual ways is part of the human experience, but creating the boundaries for what is safe and acceptable when women and men living with dementia may find it difficult to navigate those boundaries continues to be a challenge for us all. Whether you like it or will offer it yourself is something we learn about one another and then respect that preference. The alternative – to live and die without a kind touch and sensitive care and the opportunity for a hug if you would like one – is not only unimaginable, but potentially cruel. The definition for neglect and abuse in the current Safeguarding Policy for Adults at Risk is clear that withholding or not offering appropriate care and social stimulation, medication, food and drink can be considered neglectful or abusive.

As a psychology student, I was both horrified and intrigued by the social and psychological research that provides us with these conclusions. This research usually involves primates and is very sad to see, but, as our closest relatives, we can see similarities in the eyes and body language and the responses to neglect and abuse.

Textbooks and journal articles in psycho-social research are full of studies of children and adults who have become psychologically damaged through lack of caring human touch.

Caring non-sexual touch can also be easily misunderstood, especially when the information-processing capacity of the brain is affected by dementia.

Karen is helping Barry Evans with his bath. He has had a stroke and has vascular dementia. He has often commented on her figure and says, 'Your boyfriend is a lucky chap.' She says, 'I don't have a boyfriend, Barry, I don't have time.' They have always shared a joke and a laugh. As she leans over him to adjust the hoist, he fondles her breast and says, 'Ooh, lovely.' Karen pulls away and looks sternly at him. 'None of that, Barry, that's going too far. I am your care worker, not your girlfriend.'

She hands him the soap and says, 'You take care of what you can manage. I need to step out a minute.' Karen pulls the alarm cord, and her colleague Janet puts her head around the door. 'Everything OK in here?'

'Yes, I need to go to the ladies urgently. Could you please help Barry finish his bath and take him back to his room?'

Later that day Karen finds time to talk to the manager about what happened in the morning. Apparently, Barry had been touching other female staff and saying complimentary but sexually explicit things. At handover that afternoon, the manager comments that Barry seems to be missing his 'home comforts' – that as he begins to feel more comfortable at the home and with the staff, his friendliness and banter seem to be crossing a line. She asks the staff how they should work together with Barry and how they are going to address his obviously more sexual behaviour.

The staff come up with a protocol that they write into his care plan. The manager who knows him well will have coffee with him and have a chat about what he might be missing in his life and how the home can support him better. She will also make it very clear how he is to behave with the care staff. This needs to be done with clear communication, in ways that Barry will be able to understand.

Living with dementia in an unfamiliar environment with little privacy, the wrong bed, wearing pyjamas (!) and the absence of a lover (or a dog or a cat or two) can increase experiences of stress, distress, anxiety and frustration. Humans often reduce stress and increase feelings of wellbeing through sex, intimacy, masturbation or self-pleasuring. Simply not having a person or pets in the bed beside you can result in feelings of loss and abandonment, fear and vulnerability. It is also one of the few choices a person can still make about their body and their control of it as they feel pleasure and release and possibly share that with another. It increases a sense of agency and self-determination in a situation where there may be little of either.

We would also do well to consider the numerous preferences for bedtime and sleep as well as for sex and cuddling in order to provide as much comfort as possible and not to jump to conclusions about how and why people seek one another's company. When sleeping with others in the care home occurs, conversations with all concerned can often alleviate any fears or distress as long as everyone ensures that the wellbeing, safety and comfort of all the residents is at the heart of the matter. Creative and sometimes playful alternatives can be discovered if we are open and flexible.

The manager of the care home asked Joe to step into his office when he came to visit his husband Gary. He was told that Gary had been found in the beds of three of the other residents over the past week. Two were women, one was a man. Gary snuggles in and goes to sleep, and so does the other person. Bill Harrison's wife Nan was outraged when she came to visit him and Gary was lying on the bed with Bill, the two of them obviously having an after-lunch nap. She told the manager that she would not stand for this kind of thing and was appalled that he could have let it happen. 'My husband isn't that sort of man.'

After discussions in the office with the manager about dementia and the need for closeness and comfort, Mrs Harris decided it was OK 'as long as it goes no further'. She said, 'I could see that Bill was relaxed and comfortable with it. It's just a bit of a shock, that's all.'

A lengthy discussion with Joe about his and Gary's sleeping arrangements showed that not only had Gary been used to sleeping with his husband in a double bed every night for the past 25 years, but they also had at least two cats and a small dog in the bed with them. Soft animals and a favourite dressing gown were brought into the home to keep Gary company in bed. Joe frequently brought Barnie, their Westie, into the home at nap time and they both snuggled with Gary on his bed. Joe was able to bring Gary home overnight to sleep in their busy, cosy bed once a month with great success and enormous amounts of wellbeing. Gary's need to find bed buddies decreased. But it did not totally stop. No one minded. Now Barnie is occasionally invited to do the same with other residents.

Spirituality and Sexuality – Other Strange Bedfellows?

For centuries and across cultures and religions, humans have been aware of the connection between the sensual, sexual and the spiritual. Written down in poetry and prose, sacred texts such as the Song of Solomon in the Old Testament, couplets and motets, music, sculpture and painting, the hand of the Divine reaches down from heaven and blesses us with some of the most joyful, passionate and ecstatic moments of our lives. Some lovers describe ethereal, out-of-mind experiences of absolutely pure sensation and earth-shattering delight.

The Ancient Greek god Eros inspired the word for sexual and sensual attraction between people: our word 'erotic' originates here. Interestingly, the Greeks made the distinction that it was not the same as *storge*, the love one has for children and family. Eros also inspires the pursuit of the ideal of youthful or inner beauty which can lead to sexual and sensual feelings. The Greek philosopher Plato saw Eros as a spiritual embodiment of beauty and therefore the lover need not actually be physically beautiful. A 'platonic' relationship is a close relationship without sexual or erotic feelings. Plato's idea was that love could exist without sex and could transcend sex or eroticism as the purest ideal. Plato and his followers believed that it could inspire creativity that will lead to a spiritual truth. We see here that the idea of a spiritual, creative tension has ancient roots. Freud described *eros* as the first human instinct and the 'life force' upon which he based his theories of psychoanalysis. It is no mistake that some of the writings of the mystics of the Christian Church walked a fine line between the *earthly/sexual* and the spiritual, often using language reserved for sexual experiences to describe their love affair with God or Jesus Christ. The language used is predominantly the language of sexual, sensual love and we can see the origins of this interweaving of the *sexual/erotic* and the spiritual developing from the Greeks. Early Christians would replace *eros* with *agape*, the love for others and the love between God and his children, and *philia* or brotherly love and friendship, in terms of importance. The strength and power of the sexual and spiritual combination has ever been present and so the resurgence of the erotic/ecstatic experience of the early male and female Christian mystics was viewed as heretical and highly suspect. Some were imprisoned, tortured, exiled or killed for their new-found ecstatic love of God and the apparent powerful attraction and appeal that accompanied them. Words such as lover, beloved, transcendent, embraced, desire, ecstatic, ecstasy, united, blissful, sacred, rapture, delight, partner, husband, longing, joined, and the actual naming or inference of body parts – lips, eyes, arms and legs, heart, soul and genitalia – have been used to describe this intense spiritual relationship.

I continue to be aware, through my own experiences in school and church, that Catholic nuns refer to themselves as, and are called, 'Brides of Christ' and are married to Christ for life. Indeed, the ceremony of final profession of religious vows in most convents involves wearing bridal attire and receiving a wedding ring to symbolise the union.

A wonderful anthology from Daniel Landinsky (2002) entitled *Love Poems from God* brings together 'twelve sacred voices from East and West'. The language of the poetry is sensual, sacred, erotic and mystical. Often humorous, these poems create an experience of God across centuries and cultures, full of earthy language, which at the same time transports us to a place of intimate connection with God the beloved and fills the reader with a sense of wonder and wellbeing.

As with everything else we have been describing in this book, the brain is at the heart of it all, so to speak. It is from here, within this control centre, this complex interwoven web of sensation, memory, history and imagination, that all of these experiences emanate. Experiences that, in the main, create a state of wellbeing. There is a significant amount of anecdotal as well as some scientific evidence that older adults who have a faith and a community of fellow believers are generally in better health and have fewer episodes of depression. Horstman (2012) briefly describes a series of studies from the Duke University Centre for Spirituality, Theology and Health, referring to their research of almost 4000 people aged 65 or older. According to the research, the participants reported benefits of daily prayer and regular attendance at religious services. These women and men showed consistently lower blood pressure, which would reduce their risk of having a stroke. In a similar study (Koenig, George and Titus 2004), older people who attended church were hospitalised less frequently, and if they were in hospital, they recovered more quickly from depression.

Indeed, persons living with dementia are well able to experience their faith and respond appropriately to liturgy, prayers, chants, scriptures, hymns, rituals and songs throughout the experience of living with dementia. Two books that I have found especially helpful and inspirational are *Ageing and Spirituality across Faiths and Cultures* (2010) edited by Elizabeth Mackinlay and *Finding Meaning in the Experience of Dementia: The Place of Spiritual Reminiscence Work* (2012) by Mackinlay and Trevitt; both offer more specific insights on spirituality and living with dementia based on their extensive research.

Horstman (2012) also describes recent studies that show an overlap in parts of the brain that experience sex and religious feeling or God. Parts of the brain are associated with romantic love and erotic feelings. As early as the late 1800s, there was a link between religious emotionalism and epilepsy. Spiritual and religious feelings have long been associated with the use of particular drugs, illicit and prescribed. Lives have even been transformed following brain injury or surgery, into new lives of oneness with the universe, transcendence and euphoria. Today there is scepticism in some quarters between relationships with God that create ecstatic experience, visions and audible conversations and some forms of mental illness, especially schizophrenia.

Horstman reports that Andrew Newberg, a Jefferson University neuroscientist, scanned the brains of Catholic nuns at prayer and Buddhist monks during meditation. He found that the brain activity charted was the same as that for sexually aroused subjects from other research sources. 'Religious experiences produce sensations of bliss, transcendence beyond one's self and unity with the loved one that is very like the ecstasy of orgasm' (2012, p.187).

The sense of transcendence, of unity with another, 'the beloved', a higher power or God, can open our souls and bodies, via the brain, to altered states of being, some of them sensual, sexual, erotic and literally 'awesome'. Most add to our sense of wellbeing.

This is the same brain that may already be struggling to make sense of Self and the inner and outer world as dementia develops. We are reading more about mindfulness training for people living with dementia. One example is a small pilot study in 2013 by Leader and colleagues which introduces 12 people living with dementia and eight caregivers to the use of mindfulness techniques and gathers their experiences afterwards (Leader *et al.* 2014). Their research question had been to see whether mindfulness practice could improve the quality of life for the person living with dementia. The overall results are encouraging and indicate that improvements for many people can take place: they report feeling more relaxed and able to let things that previously caused stress and anxiety take more of a back seat in their daily experiences. Carers reported similar positive reactions. Further, more detailed studies are planned. Aromatherapy massage and other complementary therapies have also been used in an attempt to reduce accompanying stress or distress. Relationships, environments and activities that enhance feelings of wellbeing, be they sexual, sensual or spiritual, add to the lived experience of dementia in more positive ways than we once could have imagined.

In our holistic and person-centred approach to those living with dementia, their experiences of themselves as sexual and sensual beings may have existed in parallel with seeing and experiencing themselves as spiritual beings. Gaining a glimmer of these connections as they improve the wellbeing of some women and men living with dementia can inform and illuminate our present understanding, and add new and essential layers of meaning and appreciation for those whom we support. It is interesting that many find talking about their spirituality, which they consider a private affair, particularly difficult. In fact, many have been schooled in the age-old belief that one does not talk about sex, politics or religion in order to cause the least offence to others. Spirituality is also an area of life, as is sex, where, when an individual is less able to meet their spiritual or sexual needs on their own, others may find it a challenge to do so with them or on their behalf. As far as we know, people do not usually expire from lack of sex or spiritual life, whatever their tradition or preference may be, but we do know that the experience of both can significantly enhance the psychological and physical attributes of wellbeing.

'Mary', a woman in her 70s living with Alzheimer's disease, describes her enhanced sexual and spiritual life as a consequence of living with dementia in a chapter entitled 'Something Better' in Whitman's beautiful book *People with Dementia Speak Out* (2016). Her faith and spiritual life have deepened as well as her sexual love for her husband and their sharing of both. In summing up, Mary tells us: 'I guess that "something better" has now become a deepening discovery of love, involving both sexuality and spirituality, possible even after years of dementia' (p.245).

It is possible that we might also learn about spirituality – in its broadest sense, even in the absence of a formal religious tradition – as a means of stress reduction. Being in the beauty of the natural world, experiencing the joy of relationships, sexual and platonic, becoming more playful and spontaneous, enjoying music, dance, meditation, the creative arts, delicious food and drink, living in the moment with gratitude can all add to how we experience the 'spiritual' and can help us to release and relieve stress.

We may wish to incorporate some or more of these activities or practices into our own lives now to help reduce the various types of stress that many believe are risk factors for developing dementia.

Points for Reflection

Without judgement, but with mindful awareness and acceptance, have a look at the statements and questions below to help guide your reflections.

- » Notice your overall impression of this chapter – what does that feel like to you?

- » How do you sense your own sensuality after reading this chapter?

- » Do you have a clearer vision of the sensuality of the person living with dementia and how that might be experienced in positive ways?

- » Are there aspects of a person's behaviour that you see differently now?

- » How has this chapter informed your thinking about, and responding to, sex and the person living with dementia when misunderstanding and/or miscuing may take place?

- » How has this chapter enhanced your understanding of the sexual/spiritual connection?

- » What would you like to think/say/do differently?

- » If you support staff in your professional role, how might you engage with them around these topics?

4

Person-Centred Conversations about Sex, Dementia and Wellbeing

If we agree that most of us find conversations about sex with our elders or juniors, and especially parents or relatives, embarrassing and difficult, perhaps it would help if we created some guidelines to help the process along.

We need look no further than the person-centred approach which seems to be the sure foundation upon which our present approach to supporting those living and working with a dementia is based.

The person-centred approach originated with Carl Rogers in the 1950s, with its biggest impact on person-centred or client-centred therapy or counselling, and in particular with the publication of Rogers' seminal work *A Way of Being* (1980). Tom Kitwood's person-centred approach to dementia care has become the foundation for much excellent research, and dynamic responsive and proactive care is based on Rogers' person-centred approach to the individual.

At the heart of the person-centred relationship is our ability to offer our Self in what Rogers calls the Core Conditions (1980). These are *Empathy* or understanding from the perspective or 'perceptual world' (or internal frame of reference) of the other, *Unconditional Positive Regard* or non-judgemental acceptance, and *Congruence* or the ability to be real, consistent and genuine in the relationship.

The hope is that we can offer these conditions, which Rogers describes as 'necessary and sufficient' in a therapeutic or helpful and growthful relationship. Therapeutic is essentially a state of being that engenders trust and openness and produces a feeling of being listened to and valued or, in Rogers' term, 'prized'. Through these conditions, the persons in relationship experience a sense of wellbeing. This state allows us to take risks to work at 'relational depth' as described by Mearns and Thorne (2000) and discussed in more detail in my previous book (Lipinska 2009). Depths in emotional connection engender trust and safety and encourage sharing. We arrive at this state of offering our authentic Self in the relationship only after we have done our homework, study, reflection and supervision, and when we take our assumptions, fear, blind spots out and allow ourselves to look at their origins, appreciate the feelings we may have about them, make an informed decision to choose alternatives if we can, and then bid them adieu. For they no longer serve us well and can create barriers to authentic relationships where the idea of personhood is valued and given.

With Rogers' Core Conditions in mind, we can then see how Kitwood's philosophy, approach and models of understanding and care are so effective. The work of Kitwood and colleagues has indeed given us an alternative paradigm from which to relate to men and women living with dementia, their partners, families and the professionals who support them in their homes and communities and across nations.

For my part, further studies in the person-centred approach have offered the opportunity to review the importance of Rogers' other core theories, the Actualising Tendency and Self-Actualisation, as seen in the lives of persons living with dementia.

Rogers' well-known example of how this tendency works is described by his observation that, even in a dark basement, potatoes have a tendency to grow, given the minimum conditions. The new and determined potato shoots will grow outwards in search of light and water and soil.

Rogers and those who adopt the person-centred approach believe that this innate tendency is within us all and, given the right conditions, our goal is then to self-actualise – in effect, to become our own best and true potato, our authentic Self.

I am sure we have seen numerous occasions, in our own lives and the lives of others in far-flung countries and across history, where, against all odds, individuals survive, thrive and flourish. I see many examples of persons living with dementia, who, in spite of their neurological status, develop new ways of being and create a different narrative for themselves – one that neither they nor anyone else could have imagined. Some examples of these changes include women and men speaking about living with dementia at international conferences, advising governments, researchers and academics, creating sculptures and paintings, writing poetry, books and plays. Christine Bryden, who was diagnosed with young-onset dementia at the age of 46, describes herself as a survivor of dementia and is an advocate and activist, author and international speaker and policy advisor. Kate Swaffer, author of *What the Hell Happened to My Brain?* (2016), was diagnosed at 49 and describes herself as 'living beyond dementia'. Both women report living with loving and supportive husbands.

I have experienced these and other women and men with dementia emphatically claiming their right to be seen and heard, to move towards what they want and need in the moment or in the short term, sometimes at odds with those around them who may have different ideas. The notion of self-actualisation is the individual's striving to have their needs, goals and desires aligned to their own unique purpose, and we have much to learn.

People become single-minded in their pursuit of self-actualisation. If there is an element of disinhibition as a result of brain changes associated with dementia, then behaviour, especially with regard to intimate and sexual behaviour, is often labelled 'challenging', 'inappropriate' or 'aggressive', and becomes a 'problem' to be solved or ignored. However, we know that this is more a reflection of the observer's response rather than what may be a very real need for human contact, comfort, belonging and, sometimes, sex.

We have now come full circle to the individual's notion of what constitutes 'wellbeing' for him or her. It will not be the same for any of us. Where the idea of wellbeing, contentment, happiness, a feeling of all being well with the world, includes a satisfying sex life, then the ideas of wellbeing and self-actualisation are entwined. Our challenge – and, I would add, our privilege – is to create an appreciation and respect for our sexualities and opportunities for healthy conversations based on what we know about sex and the brain, sex and older people, sex and younger adults when cognitive changes or disability occur, within the particular context of individual sexual history and preferences – and to share our learning with others.

Back to Kitwood's Person-Centred Basics

In an effort to provide a framework or guidelines for thinking about dementia and sex and the conversations we might wish we could have, let's return to a combination of Rogers' Core Conditions and Kitwood's psychological needs of people with dementia.

Kitwood identifies these as Comfort, Identity, Attachment, Inclusion, Occupation – each one of the petals of a flower held together in the centre by Love (1997).

Love

It is no coincidence that in Rogers' later years he admitted that what he had really meant all along by UPR – Unconditional Positive Regard – was, in fact, love. Kitwood unapologetically cites Love as the centre of his flower.

Tom Kitwood also speaks of the Love that is the keystone to the psychological needs of the person with dementia. Indeed, we are all in great need of it. Perhaps it is this spirit of life and humanity that propels the individual forward into tomorrow when neurology might dictate otherwise. The spiritual lover, spiritual survivor or indeed the spiritual warrior can be seen every day in the halls of residential and nursing homes, the apartment down the street, the café on the corner (Lipinska 2009).

Comfort

Interestingly, in spite of many years of familiarity with Kitwood's book *Dementia Reconsidered*, it is only very recently during this writing endeavour that I have come across the following quotation. Kitwood is referring to 'comfort' in his cluster (flower) of psychological needs of the person living with dementia: 'The heightened sexual desire that is felt by some people with dementia may be interpreted, in part at least, as manifestations of this need' (Kitwood 1997, p.82). This very much aligns my thinking with his, at least in this one aspect of how and why we humans may seek out sexual connection with Self or other(s) and why its intensity is magnified in some persons living with dementia when *dis*comfort may be a more prevalent experience. To seek out comfort in the face of ongoing discomfort and disconnection would be a very human response, life-affirming and self-actualising.

I would also suggest, although Kitwood does not, that the key to the sexual histories, needs, desires and behaviour resides within *identity*. The multiple aspects of our identities, which include our sexual identities whether we are sexually active or not, also create the unique sexual beings we have been, that we are and could continue to be, or which could be reawakened with or without behaving sexually. This also reflects the sense of continuity and consistency Kitwood writes about here.

Identity

Our approach to understanding identity, according to Kitwood, is to bring these aspects of Self together through understanding the person's life history, which we can hold on to with, and on behalf of, the other person. By responding with empathy, we can value the person as who she or he is. He proposes that meeting one of these needs sensitively will have a knock-on effect of increasing a sense of wellbeing in all other aspects too.

We know that identity is the key to trying to understand and appreciate the whole person in the glimmer we see and that they choose to share with us. This includes their past, present *and* future. Certainly, no matter where a person is on the continuum of their experience of dementia, a future and a future identity is always there, in the next moment, just around the corner, until the final breath. I hear of many occasions of wonderful loving and supportive care at the end of life and careful, considerate preparation of persons with dementia and their families for the kind of death they may have planned or would have wished.

When we consider sexual identity, it is important that we appreciate the pervasiveness of sexuality as it influences and is influenced by all other aspects of a person's identity, and that is so much more than who they choose to love or have sex with. This quotation is a great example of what I mean:

> I think sometimes people see it as all about sex! What you do in bed I mean. If I didn't have sex at all with another woman for the rest of my life, I would still be a lesbian. It's as integral to who I am as my identity as a mother, the job that I do and the beliefs I hold dear. It's not the whole of me but it is a big part! (Knocker and Smith 2017, p.14)

When I think about my own identity, I can see how this applies: if I didn't have sex with a man for the rest of my life, I would still be heterosexual.

My concern is that we have learned well how to discover, involve and support the person's identity in so many ways, and yet, more often than not, the person's sexual identity is ignored or not even imagined.

Attachment

Our need for attachment, its theory attributed to John Bowlby (1969), describes aspects of childhood development rooted in our earliest relationships. It is another of the psychological needs identified by Kitwood. The bonds and attachments we form in those early years affect our relationship building and our sense of Self and trust in others. These foundations are shaken when we face threat or uncertainty and are put to the test. Most of us develop reassuring bonds resulting in secure attachments based on our experiences with parents/caregivers and a broader reliable environment in early life. Insecure and fragile attachments may create greater insecurities in some. My long career as a therapist supports my experience with clients that most often we are all on a continuum of insecurity and security over our lifetimes and over certain events.

The styles of attachment established earlier in life will ultimately influence our responses and coping styles. How we respond to change and threats to our status quo differs depending on where we might be developmentally, or the things that happen to us all in Western culture, across the life span. Some of the expected developmental tasks of ageing can induce anxieties and concerns that take us back to the quality and frequency of those earlier attachments.

When you add to this stage of development the multiple changes and losses associated with healthy ageing, you see great strength and adaptability in the coping abilities of the two generations of older adults. For the person with young-onset dementia, their developmental issues may be to do with their effectiveness in their career, their support of older parents or relatives, or their teenage or young adult children, preparing for their future and their own, including retirement and becoming grandparents.

Talking about his young-onset dementia, Ben highlights his own particular developmental challenges:

This is impossible. I've been caring for my dad – he's got all his marbles, but has gone to bits since his wife Susan died from cancer two years ago. He can't manage at the flat in London and the golf timeshare they had in Florida. How am I supposed to sort him out, and the kids still need me, even though they are both away at uni. My wife and I split up ten years ago. She remarried. I'm on my own. Who is there for me now I have this? It's ridiculous at this stage in my life. Good thing I'm self-employed. I'd die of embarrassment having to deal with this at an office somewhere.

It was pretty grim for Ben for a while, but he made friends at a men's support group for other men living with dementia. Ben and his father and the girls had a good last golfing trip together in Florida and put the apartment there up for sale. His daughters proved valuable and understanding allies.

The uncertainties and anxieties associated with changing brain function, as in dementia, can throw a curve ball at our usual coping abilities wherever we find ourselves along the developmental timeline. Our underlying appreciation of attachment can inform our decision making and planning around daily life and sharing the kinds of relationships that increase a feeling of security and safety. The panic and sense of fear that can ensue does not respond to logic and is extremely upsetting to the person themselves and those who love them and live with them.

Kate cared for her husband, George, who lived with moderate Alzheimer's disease. She described being unable to even go off to the toilet as it would create a 'catastrophic reaction' in her husband. He would continually shout for her and bang on the bathroom door until she reappeared. With support from the group to make the decision and the arrangements, George began attending the day centre for three mornings a week. Kate was better able to cope as she had some time to herself and knew that George was getting stimulation and socialisation on his terms. George became attached to one or two of the staff, which was not a problem at all. They were able to spend time with George and helped him to begin a life story book and reminisce about his favourite baseball team in the past and enjoy them in the present, on television and in magazines with photographs of players and collecting memorabilia. This was a very positive experience for George and Kate, although it didn't change George's behaviour once he was home again.

In the care home or domiciliary care setting, we might be tempted to schedule a particular member of staff as a key worker for a person with dementia, especially if they get along well. However, we must allow for the potential devastation that could ensue when that caregiver is on leave or off for the weekend. It is also easy for a well-intentioned care worker to become overly burdened and become burned out as a result. It would be best to nurture secure attachments with a small number of people who can easily overlap and fit into the day-to-day life of a person living with dementia whether at home or in a caring community.

I have long observed some individuals with dementia display an increased need for attachment in a world of unpredictable and ongoing change, much of which is anxiety-provoking.

In terms of the need for attachment and supporting people with dementia, much has now been observed and published. Apart from caring and loving relationships, many have found that doll therapy has had a positive influence on reducing the anxiety, distress and searching that is the opposite of what happens when we have strong attachments and means of meeting those needs ourselves. There has been some controversy around this form of therapy, but, having seen it in action, I am convinced of its merits. I will also freely admit that I have had a travel buddy for many years. He is a small cuddly teddy bear that accompanies me on my many work trips. He is not a favourite with my husband, so is relegated to the night stand when I am at home.

I have bought many soft toys for adult friends over the years when they have been in especial need of comfort. All have been welcomed and well loved, and those friends in turn have done the same for like-minded others in their circle. Just as I know the people who will respond to such a gift from me, care staff will know which residents, women and men, will respond positively. If the therapy is available for a person to choose to pick the doll up or not, then I believe it is a matter of freedom of choice. As long as there is no pretence that this is a real 'baby' from the professional side, the person with dementia may describe the doll as a baby, a thing, the name of their own child, sister, parent, family cat, a staff member or whoever. The doll becomes a means of enhancing communication and identifying with emotion. It is interesting that when there is an equal selection of soft toy animals and dolls, the dolls are seen as the most popular choice. Gary Mitchell's recent book *Doll Therapy in Dementia Care: Evidence and Practice* (2016) is an excellent consolidation of aspects of attachment theory in practice as they improve the lived experience of persons with dementia in care homes.

I believe we can attempt to meet the individual's need for attachment by maintaining and creating authentic and reliable relationships that can anticipate the potential upset created by yet another change, or respond by upholding a person's ability to adapt appropriately if given the correct tools and support to do so. I believe that healthy attachment is also about being able to let go of relationships when they are no longer responsive to or supportive of our own developmental process. See Luke Tanner's excellent chapter on 'A Sense of Touch and the Experience of Attachment' in his book *Embracing Touch in Dementia Care: A Person-Centred Approach to Touch and Relationships* for a detailed, but easy-to-grasp, explanation of the theory in relation to touch, with examples of the experience of the person living with dementia and those who support them. He summarises by saying:

> A person's attachment style can be as much a determinant of their quality of life as their level of dementia. Understanding these different attachment styles can help care workers make sense of some very difficult, confusing and sometimes extremely distressing behaviours. (2017, p.71)

Inclusion

Kitwood describes this as our need to be included in social situations and in society at large, given that we are essentially made for group and face-to-face living. We have developed significantly in this area. We have learned from people living with dementia, who have graciously and generously included us in *their* lives and *their* world, what this means from their perspective. Our notion of custodial care and what we *thought* was good for people living with dementia has fallen short of the mark indeed.

We are learning what inclusion truly means and are still adjusting to the turned tables. Some of us are still struggling. Inclusion that creates wellbeing is that which takes into account how it is relevant to the person with dementia, their relationships and communities, how they engage with the world. Person-centred occupational therapists and activities coordinators have shared outstanding care practices in numerous journal articles and books which invite us to think deeply and act inclusively in ways that reflect the individual within the group or community. I wonder what Tom Kitwood would say about our 'dementia-friendly' places of worship, shops, banks, cafés and communities. My local Cinema City has film screenings once a month especially for persons with dementia, their families, carers and friends, with refreshments and a comfort break – cinema made easy and accessible.

When I think about 'inclusion' and sex and dementia, this means also being inclusive of the past and present sexuality and sexual identity of the person and how that might be included in living their life with dementia. It also means how that person continues to include their sexual self in their own life and their future, and whether they are interested in sexual activities or not. It means that I include their sexual self in my conversations and in my attitudes and approach and my philosophy of support and care and how I model and share that with others.

Occupation

For Kitwood, this means being involved in one's life process in personally significant ways, drawing on one's abilities and interests and sense of agency. To affirm a person's desire to be actively involved in their day-to-day lives and maintain their interests and hobbies without being patronised is quite a skill.

Kitwood says: 'The more that is known of a person's past and particularly their deepest sources of satisfaction, the more likely it is that a solution will be found' (1997, p.83). As already expressed, sexual behaviour, alone or with others, is high on many people's lists of a 'deep source of satisfaction' – an apt description. We also know that what feels good is worth repeating, remembering, storing and then retrieving for the next time. You will recognise how complex that process actually is in terms of brain function. Memories with a strong emotional connection are also remembered far longer than simple facts. The emotional components of the memories of sex and love-making may embed these particular memories in the brain for longer than the memory required to make an omelette or mow the lawn.

'Agency' – or the ability to be aware that I can get a response from someone or the environment and have an effect on what happens in the world – is a very lasting, strong and determined force. I have written elsewhere about my sense that sex may be one of the few areas of agency and control still left to a person as dementia progresses. Being able to engage in one's sex life or to put it to bed, so to speak, on one's own terms is included in the notion of agency. Sex forms a significant part of our satisfying and meaningful occupation as humans.

Creating a Person-Centred Sexual Profile

From a person-centred perspective, imagine that we are going to offer Rogers' Core Conditions of Empathy, Unconditional Positive Regard (acceptance) and Congruence to the person we are speaking to and also to ourselves. Yes, to ourselves.

This is key to making it across the potential barrier of embarrassment, discomfort and anxiety housed in knowledge deficits that may accompany this intimate topic.

If we can be understanding and caring of our own sexual selves, accepting and non-judgemental of our past, present and future, our own knowledge deficits and limitations, if we are willing to be genuine and consistent, we may be further along the path to having a meaningful conversation than we would be without this preparation. We will also be better informed and prepared for whatever reaction and response that comes back to us from the person we are speaking with. We can remain centred and calm, caring yet factual, understanding and empathic.

By mapping a person's sexuality on to Kitwood's 'flower' of psychological needs, we have a template to help us create an actual person-centred sexual profile from which can flow an actual conversation. All of us, whether we are living with dementia or not, share these needs, and their presence in our lives enhances the opportunities for us all to live well and feel affirmed and valued. In this sense, we are familiar with and can easily construe what would make these conversations work.

We can perhaps envisage now how our own thoughts and feelings can be ordered in informed and life-affirming ways, encouraging us to see the whole human being in their context. We can then use what we have learned as our point of departure for developing conversations, supporting solutions and, ultimately, co-creating life histories and plans for care. The ideal would be: 'As the whole of the cluster of needs is met, it is likely that there will be an enhancement of the global sense of self-worth of being valuable and valued' (Kitwood 1997, p.84).

We are moving together towards an increase in the sense of wellbeing.

I can hear you saying that this kind of thing requires trust and confidentiality, and it takes time to develop this kind of trust. And so it does. And yet, as previously stated, we are usually able to gather information about equally sensitive and private matters regarding finances, bowel habits and religious affiliations at a first meeting or assessment.

Here are some examples of how person-centred conversations might go:

Michelle

D: Hi, Michelle, I'm Danuta, and we spoke last week about joining our support group for younger women living with dementia. How are you feeling about it now?

M: Oh, OK, I think. I'm not sure about groups.

D: Is it something special about being in a group you aren't sure of, Michelle?

M: Well, I've never really been a group kind of person. I'm more of a loner, I think. Or maybe just being with one or two close friends or my partner, Richard.

D: Yes, you're more comfortable with one or two close people you know?

M: Yes, that's it. I won't know anyone there.

D: That's true, but you know me a little bit, and I'll be there and keeping things going.

M: Oh, right.

D: Other women at the group will also have memory problems and other challenges too.

M: Will they have Alzheimer's like I do?

D: Yes, a couple of them will. Others will have different kinds of dementia. Some will have memory and other changes.

M: What will we do? What will we talk about?

D: Well, the group is for all of you, and we can talk about whatever you want to talk about. We begin with coffee or tea and biscuits and chat a bit. How we are, how's the weather, what have we been up to. Just being sociable...

M: OK, I can manage that much.

D: Then we talk about how things have been going for everyone since we met. The group meets every two weeks.

M: Will I have to talk, take a turn?

D: No one is made to talk if they don't want to. No one is put on the spot. Most women want to share and to listen. See how they are getting along. All kinds of topics come up. Things that are affected by having dementia. What people are struggling with or doing quite well or better than expected. Relationships with partners, family, fun times...

M: Oh, right. Well, that might be good for me. I think Richard and I are driving each other crazy. I do things I don't seem to be aware of, and he gets cross and irritated with me. Sometimes he shouts. It's not like him, so I must be really messing up to make him like that. He always apologises and feels bad. He says he knows it's not my fault. Then we make up and that's always good. (*Looks sad and off into the distance. After a pause she continues.*) We're not as close as we once were. I know that bothers him more than me at the moment.

D: So things are different between you in some ways? (*Michelle nods, looking down and fidgeting with her handbag on her lap.*) You say you aren't as close as you once were, Michelle. I'm sort of reading between the lines here – please correct me if I get it wrong…do you mean in your private life, your sex life?

M: Yeah – it used to be great, and then it was just OK, and recently it's been hardly ever. But I suppose all couples go through stages. Now we are grandparents, I suppose it's bound to change, isn't it? It's not like when we first got together. It can't be, can it?

You can see from this exchange that Michelle is quite shy and reserved. As the conversation progresses, she begins to relax and become more comfortable. By the end of the conversation, she is asking for reassurance, permission to talk about it.

Which we did, in great detail, including how to help her physical symptoms and emotional state of mind, how things were before being diagnosed, what she hoped for herself now and later. And we talked about Ann Summers shops, their discreet displays and selections of adult sex toys and aids, and online suppliers that could send discreetly packaged goods to her home.

Jim

D: Jim, I know not everyone is comfortable talking about their private life, their love life, but you did tell me that you and Pat had a great marriage and you still love each other very much.

J: Love at first sight – 58 years ago.

D: I wonder if you would mind if we talked about this for a few minutes now so that we can be sure that we support you and Pat to be as close as you would like while she is living here. (*Jim nods, looking shy.*) We've talked about many aspects of Pat's life and yours as a couple and a family too. I have an idea of the things she likes and doesn't like, the things she wants to get on with herself and some things she might like some assistance with. Some of the ways dementia affects people is in their relationships and how their sex lives might change too. Now, married as long as you have been, I imagine your need and desire for closeness may not have totally disappeared. (*Jim smiles, looks down, slightly embarrassed.*) Am I right, Jim? (*Jim looks up and smiles.*) So, what can we do to help you have privacy and comfort without any interruptions or feelings of awkwardness?

J: Well, for a start, I don't want people going around saying, 'Oh they've got the door shut, we know what they're up to in there.' We might not be up to anything, but we like to hug and kiss and cuddle. You can't do that in the lounge here.

D: No, you're right. That might cause a stir. (*Both smiling.*) But I hope we would all be grown up about it. You wouldn't be the subject of gossip, Jim; we respect the residents and their families. Everyone is entitled to privacy, singles or couples, so you wouldn't be unusual.

J: Well, that's a relief. I don't want us to be a laughing stock.

D: We would do whatever feels right for you and Pat. We can give you both dinner together in her room once in a while, so you have the whole evening to yourselves. How does that sound?

J: Yeah, that's a good start. Can I bring wine?

D: Sure, Jim. Sounds lovely. Bring in your favourite glasses too. We can keep them in Pat's room.

Marion

Marion was a single professional – 'I'm the real girl about town' – with lots of friends, admirers and a great social life. She has been diagnosed with young-onset Alzheimer's disease. She told me she enjoys the online dating scene but never wanted to marry, in spite of several proposals.

D: I wonder how it's feeling now that you have had a diagnosis?

M: One of the scary things is that I'll get to the stage where I'm not as free to come and go. What if I get lost? I won't be able to go out as often as I used to, meet up with friends out of the blue for drinks or remember how to go online…meet a new date.

Marion was ready and willing to talk and had been afraid that she would never have the chance. Being single but sexual was important to Marion, and she was very able to take care of herself. She was concerned that she might betray her body by not being able to give it what it wanted, what it was used to. That meant both with lovers and self-pleasuring.

M: What if I forget how to do it? Or I forget who I'm doing it with? What if I call him the wrong name? How awful would that be?

D: You're afraid you won't remember how to do it? Or call your lover by someone else's name? I can hear the panic in your voice as you say that and see the worry in your eyes, Marion.

M: Well, you can't blame me – it's a big deal!

D: Yes, it is. Your brain and body are likely to remember how to do it for a while. Especially if there is someone helping you along. As long as you remember how to take care of yourself, your body is likely to respond.

M: So I won't forget all at once? I've got some time to figure this out. Like how to remember where I've put the batteries...but that's always been a challenge! (*Marion laughs and I smile.*)

We talked about this at length. We discussed keeping herself safe when going out alone and making sure someone she trusted knew where she was going, when and if she would be back that night. We looked at the possibility of making sure she had ID on her at all times.

M: How do you tell a lover that you have this thing? That will be the last time you see him, for sure. I don't want anyone to 'be with' on a permanent basis, I never have, and now, worst of all, to watch me go downhill. I would hate that!

To tell or not to tell? This was going to require thought and consideration on her part.

Clarity of purpose is also key to the success of person-centred conversations. It will be important to the person in conversation with you that you have the answers to some particular questions in the hope of engendering mutual respect, trust and confidence.

I have found it helpful to explore these questions from the perspective of the other person and then be able to use the answers to create sensitive communication and a feeling of safety right from the beginning.

Here are some questions that might begin to create a framework for thinking before we speak:

Do you already have a sexuality policy in place?

What does it include? Can I have a copy and can you explain it to me?

Why do you want to gather this information?

Who is going to see this information?

Who will you talk to about this information?

What will you do with this information?

What is the extent of confidentiality I can expect?

Can I specify with whom you share this information?

Can I change my mind at any time about what I have shared with you today?

Can I ask you to have conversations with others on my behalf?

How do I know you are going to respect my wishes?

How will you act in a situation where I might be the victim of sexual threat, harm or abuse?

What will you do if I am unaware of my own behaviour which might be sexually threatening, harmful or abusive towards others?

Could these questions and answers create a helpful backdrop to how we then proceed?

The questions are not to be asked directly, but are rather guides to what we need to prepare ahead of time and know the answers to, so that they can be offered as part of the conversation if need be.

How can we support others through person-centred conversations that might lead to an experience of wellbeing?

Points for Reflection

Without judgement, but with mindful awareness and acceptance, have a look at the statements and questions below to help guide your reflections.

» Notice your overall impression of this chapter – what does that feel like to you?

» Has your understanding of the person-centred approach been enhanced by this chapter or has it stayed the same?

» How useful was refocusing Kitwood's psychological needs of persons with dementia through a sexual lens?

» How might what you have learned here support you to think/say/do things differently?

» If you support staff in your professional role, how might you engage with them around these topics?

5

Explorations through Training

In the very early days, back in New Hampshire, USA, I began a series of lectures for postgraduate nurses on the subject of adult sexuality in later life. One courageous nurse in an early group described this actual dilemma as she experienced it:

> I have worked with older people for most of my career as a nurse, and I always thought I was open and approachable and not bound by stereotypical thinking. This workshop has reminded me how deep-seated my prejudice is when it comes to my own parents. Recently I went to visit my 78-year-old widowed mother with the kids. I went into the bedroom to put our coats on the bed, and the twin beds that my parents had for years were gone. Something was wrong. I was initially confused and then surprised to be confronted by a queen-sized double with matching frills and cushions. I came into the kitchen while the kids were outside and asked, 'So, Mom, where are the twin beds?'
>
> I was really shocked, and even more so by how I felt.

'First of all, it's really none of your business, and second of all, I met a lovely man at tennis (said with a twinkle in her eyes), and the twin beds just weren't helpful.' After I regained my composure, we laughed and hugged, and I was truly able to say, 'Good for you, Mom.'

This example brought a deep and honest discussion in the room concerning our perceptions of how open we all believed we were about sexuality in later life. Many of us, like the nurse above, were surprised at how our attitudes changed when we thought about our own parents or grandparents as individual adults with the right to a sexual past, present and future. We spoke about our own children's views of our sexuality and had a good laugh about what they said and believed. On a more serious note, we then contemplated the notion of double standards across generations, and the reason for the incest taboo in Western culture. We explored ways of confronting our own blind spots and imagining how we could create opportunities for similar discussions with our families and work colleagues who supported older adults. In effect, we had also begun the process of advocacy for others and our own futures as older adults.

A significant part of this book has been influenced by the many training programmes I have taught, variously entitled 'Healthy Ageing', 'Adult Sexuality in Later Life' and 'Person-Centred Responses to Living Well with Dementia and Sexuality'. I am indebted to the women and men who have attended these courses in the USA and the UK from the mid-1980s to the present day. Their courageous and honest sharing has been and continues to be enlightening and encouraging.

I certainly know this has been part of my own journey over the years with numerous clients, care staff across the health and social care spectrum, and women and men living with dementia or caring for them, which has culminated in the writing of this book.

When I reflect on these many courses and groups of up to 18 in any given course, my experience has been primarily from the heteronormative perspective. Very few in the groups have ever shared their own sexual identities or preferences. Occasionally, women and men have shared concerns for their own ageing and identity and the possible development of dementia. I was pleased one day to have a chat with a woman participant who came to me at the break and identified herself as queer and said that she was grateful to have felt included and welcomed in the course, and that this was not her usual experience. Responses to the exercise below will highlight important differences, nuance and language – as well as many similarities – if the participants were LGBTQI people. There have been many more articles, projects, books and training programmes produced to better reflect our diverse lifestyles in the 21st century, but we still have more to do together.

I have reproduced here some of the exercises that have formed part of the training programmes in an effort to introduce you to a means of becoming more familiar with the topic and to encourage you to use them in whatever way you might find helpful.

I have referenced a few other training tools which are excellent in my view: namely, *The Last Taboo* (2011) from Sally Bamford and the International Longevity Centre; *Dementia Care Matters Module Eleven: A Kiss is Still a Kiss* (2016); and Sally Knocker's resource *Safe to Be Me* from

Age UK (Knocker and Smith 2017). See References for full details.

It may be helpful to have a few tools at hand to be able to reflect on our innermost thoughts and feelings as we go through this book, and, if we are honest, to gain a real sense of where our blind spots may be (we all have them) and how to get past them so we can be open and welcoming to the concerns or celebrations of others.

I encourage you to use and share these as you wish.

Here is an example of some of the questions to get us started in our discussions.

Several of the questions are answered throughout this text. I have given an overview of some of the answers to questions 3, 4, part of 5, and 11.

Things to consider:

1. My own and others' attitudes towards sexuality in older people and those with dementia, ageism, stereotypes, discrimination, values, faith, spirituality, gender, sexual preferences and identity, culture, legal status and the law.

2. Biological imperatives: eat, drink, eliminate, copulate, sleep.

3. Why do people have sex? (This is usually rephrased as '*If* people have sex' – as not all adults do – 'why do they?')

4. What do we do when we can't?

5. Sexual history, gender, identity and sexual preference. What are our thoughts and feelings about, and relationships with, lesbian, gay, bisexual, trans, queer and intersex and asexual (LGBTQI) men and women,

hidden sexuality? What happens when these people also develop dementia?

6. Sexuality/sensuality/intimacy? Same or different?

7. How is the need for sex and intimacy affected by dementia? Brain and behaviour?

8. How might the 'sexual taboo' interfere with seeing adults with dementia as men and women with rights and needs, thoughts and feelings?

9. The role of the Human Rights Act, Mental Capacity Act, consent, safeguarding policies and procedures.

10. The role of bereavement, loss and grief around sexuality, partners and sexual identity.

11. Sex as energy, identity, communication, wellbeing, celebration.

12. How can a person-centred approach be used to value sex and dementia with a view to enhancing wellbeing?

With question 3, I invite the group to say whatever they know to be true and not to censor themselves in any way. I am sure you can add to the list yourself. We need to be mindful that the list will also be different if we are working with mixed cultural groups, genders and ages.

It is always fascinating to note that, invariably, procreation or 'to have children' is not at the top of any list. Often it is somewhere in the middle of the page of flipchart paper. On one occasion, reproduction was nearly at the bottom. The location of this word gives rise to an interesting discussion. I believe that it would leap to the top of the list, along with love, if participants were of our parents' or grandparents' generation.

The list can include but is not limited to:

it feels good

to get a promotion

peer pressure

to keep a job

it's a good stress reliever

to keep a secret

it's (usually) free fun

anger/revenge

rite of passage

to keep a lover

exploration

to experiment

curiosity

to push my boundaries

to get it over with

reward

punishment

to have children

to show love and affection

fear

to be in control

lust

to take risks

to earn a living

to be naughty

to discredit someone else/get them in trouble

to gain a reputation

to be noticed/appreciated

be good at something

to pay for drugs/booze/food/rent/clothes

to stay in a flat/house

do what is expected by parents/culture

to piss off the parents/establishment

pity

force a relationship break-up

adultery or two-timing

can do it on my own

to be close	to have influence
reaffirm my identity	for enjoyment and pleasure
to feel attractive/desired	
intimacy	to go to great places before
warmth and cuddles	boredom

In addition to the list above, there followed an exploration of some of the physical benefits of sex. Although these benefits are available for most of us, we can imagine that, for older adults, those benefits could be more than helpful towards general health, and overall often lead to a more general improved sense of wellbeing.

These benefits included increased appetite, longer and deeper sleep, reduced blood pressure and increased cardiovascular activity; reduced stress and anxiety and increased relaxation and vitality; increased mobility and flexibility; increased digestive motility and reduced constipation – to name the most common. The kind of exercise associated with sex is deemed to be healthy and desirable in more ways than the obvious. In addition, Dr Dayu Lin of the NYU Langone Medical Center (cited in Long 2014) is only one neuroscientist of many across the globe working on the belief that having sex has a positive influence (at least in rodents) on the development of brain cells in the hippocampus, which plays a vital role in memory. It is possible that the death of brain cells that leads to memory loss associated with dementia may be minimised. So, having sex is not only good for us emotionally, physically, spiritually and socially, but our brains like it too.

Further questions and answers give us insight into the human condition and the ways in which we can cope and learn to defer sexual gratification. It would be safe to assume that most sexually active adults will have had to learn the art of mastery over their libido during a lifetime. It would be reasonable to assume that some of those behaviours would be shared and similar to our peers. If that is so, then we have on hand a repertoire of potential activities that have been tried and tested as alternatives to sex. Some may work better than others for different people and for different reasons. Knowing the life story of those we support and having conversations with them and/or their partners (if they have them) about alternatives they have found helpful could be invaluable.

Here are some examples:

What do people do when they can't have sex (if it's inconvenient or inappropriate)?

phone a friend

masturbate in private

do the housework

meditate/pray

take a cold shower/bath

phone sex

go to the gym

sexting

take the dog for a walk

cybersex

watch an adult movie

sex chat room

do the gardening/mow the lawn

eat

read a sexy novel

drink

do drugs/smoke dope

bake/cook

get a massage

pedicure/manicure

play computer games

kick boxing

smoke

go to the pub

play sports

cry

get depressed

make sure it's great when you can

arrange to go away with lover

arrange for kids to go away

leave work early to meet a lover

meet at lunch time for a quickie

become a monk

get your own place/ leave parental home

take a nap

take a pill

do the decorating

not 'out' so it's tricky

Not only does a list like this invite laughter and honesty, but it also encourages a deeper and more serious discussion of some of the more upsetting reasons why sex might not be possible in the short term or in the future. Tears are also not unusual during this exercise as people reflect on their own and others' sexual histories and absent lovers or loss of interest.

When we reflect on this list, we can see that most sexually active adults will create alternatives to having sex when they might want to. We have learned to postpone gratification. They create diversions which combine taking their minds off it and building up and release in physical energy, enough to make them feel satisfied and expended/tired afterwards.

When we consider women and men living with dementia, either in their own homes or in community living, we might now have a better understanding of what might be helpful to them if they find they are unable to have sex if and when they want to. As we have *learned* to postpone sexual gratification, that learning relies on memory to be able to put these alternatives in place. It may not be as easy as it once was to call to mind how to do that and extract oneself from an embarrassing and possibly dangerous situation. This may give rise to occasions when sexual behaviour and/or verbalised thoughts and feelings become an out-loud and visible extension of the individual in the here and now. By expanding our knowledge of alternatives to sex that might be helpful, we might be able to protect that person's dignity and privacy, and that of others in the immediate environment.

To be person-centred in our approach also means acknowledging what we hear and see in the here and now, yet keeping ourselves and others safe; and then calmly and quickly offering options to ensure dignity, privacy and an alternative activity that will use energy and give a positive feeling of pleasure and enjoyment. This requires us as professionals to have had training to appreciate this set of circumstances and be able to engage in conversations with persons with dementia and/or their partners or family.

Sexual history can include but is not limited to:

childhood sexual abuse: victim/perpetrator	war crimes of a sexual nature
sexual abuse	FGM (female genital mutilation)
pregnancy	
abortion	prostitution: men, women, children
miscarriage	sex trafficking: victim/perpetrator
lost paternity (see below)	
infanticide	sexual harassment and sexual offences
rape: victim/perpetrator	

orgies

one-night stands

sexual addiction

pornography

paedophilia

voyeurism

internet/phone sex/ sexting

chat rooms

multiple partners

S&M

friends, partners, family and children lost to HIV/AIDS

cross dressing/drag

LGBTQI sex and asexuality

celibacy

ritualised sex and Satanism

incest/abuse

enforced childhood marriage

And all the possible places and ways to have sex known to humans since time began.

This is by no means an exclusive list, but is based on those issues I have encountered with participants in training programmes, or with clients in counselling or in consultations across various care environments.

An example of lost paternity

Pointing to the visitors going into his neighbour's room in the care home, Jim asked me one day, 'Is that man Bernie's son?' I explained that he was, and that he was here with his daughters to visit his father, their grandfather. Jim's eyes brimmed with tears, and he grabbed my hand, gesturing with his head for me to sit down. 'I had one of those once,' he said almost in a whisper.

'Did you, Jim?' I wasn't entirely sure what he meant, but he did go on to tell me about Sadie, the love of his life. They were both 16. Sadie became pregnant, and they were terrified, poor, shocked and thrilled. It was quite the scandal. Jim was sent to work with a distant cousin in his garage in Wales. Sadie was sent away to an aunt in Scotland to have the baby. He never knew how to find her or what happened to her or the baby. 'She disappeared.' But somewhere in the world there was probably a child of his who by now also probably had their own family. Like Bernie.

The tears were freely flowing as Jim recounted his painful losses. He had never married or had children. 'Not a day goes by that I don't think about both of them. But this is the first time I've talked about it.'

I thanked Jim for sharing with me, and I was very moved myself. I asked Jim if there was anything we could do together. He didn't want everyone to know. After talking for a while, he decided to create a birthday for his child and chose a name that could be for a girl or a boy. He asked if we could get a video on Scotland. He didn't want to read any more, he said, but a video would be good. 'It makes it more real to me. And at least someone knows. It's a weight lifted off my shoulders, I can tell you.'

This encounter was extremely important for me too. I had known older women who had lost lovers, mourned lost babies, but I honestly had not thought about lost paternity and the role it played in a man's life, especially towards the end of his life. If he developed dementia, there was a high probability that no one might ever know. It increased my sensitivity around men's life histories and ways to make it possible for them to introduce a subject if they wanted to, knowing that it was safe to do so and they would not be judged. At the same time, I knew that it was a secret that many would not wish to share. Knowing that it was a possibility enhanced my appreciation for the possibility and allowed me to open others to the same, through introducing it as a point of raising awareness in training.

Through ongoing and relevant training, we can learn together and appreciate this rarely discussed topic in new ways to influence those around us and those whom we support to recognise that sexuality is part of all of our lives. We can become informed advocates for sexual rights and choice for women and men, irrespective of age or diagnosis, gender or sexual identity. In effect, in so doing, we also become good advocates for ourselves and our own ageing and the possibility of living with dementia as still sexual and sensual beings.

Points for Reflection

Without judgement, but with mindful awareness and acceptance, have a look at the statements and questions below to help guide your reflections.

» Notice your overall impression of this chapter – what does that feel like to you?

» What was it like to imagine people you support from the perspective of reasons why people may engage in sex? Were you able to add any more reasons?

» How did you relate to the list of what people might do when they are unable to have sex? Did you add some other things to do?

» What was your response to the scenario describing lost paternity?

» Has your understanding of the history of the person living with dementia been enhanced by this chapter or has it stayed the same?

» How might what you have learned here support you to think/say/do things differently?

» If you support staff in your professional role, how might you engage with them around these topics?

» Has this chapter inspired you to look for other training tools, courses or methods to help your own learning and that of staff you may support?

Conclusion

We have now arrived at the end of the book.

I hope that there have been some thoughtful moments, support and encouragement to live your best and whole Self, including the breadth and depth and precious individuality of your sexual and sensual Self. It is the only one we have, after all.

Perhaps you have been affirmed in your way of being and how you support and encourage others to find meaning and expression in their sexuality and sensuality, irrespective of age and/or diagnosis or brain function.

Above all, I hope that you may go forward in the knowledge that if we are courageous and work together for change, sensitivity and inclusion, all of our lives will be enriched and enhanced.

We are told that love makes the world go round. And sex will add some sparkle on the way.

Afterword

It is rare to read a book where you feel that you have been in a very deep and meaningful conversation with its author, as if you have been invited into their living room to chew the cud together and contemplate the joys and complexities of life and love. This is how I felt when reading Danuta's book, which hopefully has been your experience too. Her wisdom and tender humanity compellingly draw us in to reflect with her on this vitally important topic. This is refreshingly *not* your average dementia book! I love the fact that this is not about people living with dementia as somehow different or separate, it is a book about *all of us* and what it means to be vibrant sexual and sensual beings in this sometimes troubled but always beautiful world of ours. Danuta talks at the beginning of holding 'two voices' in our heads, 'being mindful of past trauma, the need to prevent harm and abuse, to celebrate difference and desire, we can also give equal voice and place for sex and intimacy in the lives of men and women living with dementia'. I think this book is a vitally important and timely start to redress the balance in the dementia care world where so much of the time sexuality is only talked about when it is perceived as a 'problem' rather than a fundamental part of our wellbeing.

As a lesbian woman, who struggled in my early life with many negative perceptions of who I was, in my middle-aged life and as my responsibilities as a mother change, I enjoy a greater confidence in both body and spirit to be comfortable and safe to really be me. I am a person who is flirtatious and cheeky with both genders and I would very much hope to see that as something that might be included and nurtured as a core part of my identity in my care plan if I were to develop a dementia. As Danuta says, 'Love makes the world go round, we are told, and so does flirting!' At a more profound level the expression of our sexuality and sensuality taps into our core needs as humans to be cherished and to cherish others, to be held and to hold another as a way of affirming being alive, even and perhaps especially when our cognitive abilities are diminishing and letting us down. Of course the expression of sexual pleasure is not necessarily with another person. I remember being momentarily disconcerted or shocked even when I was asked to help write a risk assessment for a vibrator for a 102-year-old woman living in a care home. Yet on reflection I challenged my own ageism in my reaction, and was delighted that the enlightened care team were looking for ways to support this woman to still enjoy the energy and release of orgasm right till the last days of her life. And when we really think about it, why ever not? In my book, it certainly beats Bingo and baking.

So why then is this a conversation that so many are neglecting to have with individuals themselves, with partners and family members and with colleagues in team meetings, supervision and training? Far too often the excuse is given that it is too intrusive or personal a subject matter. Many of us are embarrassed or awkward because these are the messages we have received in our own upbringings about sex being a taboo topic. Yet in my experience when we are brave enough to open these conversations, there is huge relief and often powerful revelations and insights to be shared as Danuta's many stories in this book reveal. Danuta also invites us to reflect on what we do when we can't have sex, or the things we do to create sensuality in our lives; these are incredibly important things to know about individuals when thinking about wellbeing, but are very unlikely to be part of any standard care assessments. There were also fascinating insights into the importance of sensory memory and how little we pay attention to how touch, taste, sound and smell can all tap into our past experiences of love and desire.

I see this book as a call to action to us all to be brave and true and steadfast in our inclusion of questions of sexuality and intimacy in all we do to further the wellbeing of people living with dementia, whatever our roles. 'Nobody's business' is often used as everybody's excuse, but none of us can finish reading this book without undertaking to *make it* our business to follow Danuta's inspiring lead and start our own conversations. As she says, 'Who knows where this may lead? Perhaps we won't find the answers yet, but staying open to questions invites openness and that allows room for the creative and the spiritual.'

Amen to that.

Sally Knocker
Consultant Trainer, Dementia Care
Matters and Opening Doors London
Rainbow Memory Cafe Coordinator

Bibliography

Amthor, F. (2012) *Neuroscience for Dummies.* Mississauga, ON: John Wiley & Sons Canada.

Archibald, C. (1994) 'Never too late to fall in love.' *Journal of Dementia Care 2,* 5, 20–21.

Baker, C. (2015) *Developing Excellent Care for People Living With Dementia in Care Homes* (University of Bradford Good Practice Guides). London: Jessica Kingsley Publishers.

Bamford, S. (2011) *The Last Taboo: A Guide to Dementia, Sexuality, Intimacy and Sexual Behaviour in Care Homes.* London: International Longevity Centre. Available at www.ilcuk.org.uk/files/pdf_pdf_184. pdf (accessed 26 June 2017).

Bowlby, J. (1969) *Attachment and Loss. Volume 1: Attachment.* London: Hogarth Press.

Brizendine, L. (2010) *The Male Brain.* London: Bantam Press.

Brooker, D. (2006) *Person-Centred Dementia Care: Making Services Better.* London: Jessica Kingsley Publishers.

Dementia Today (2013) 'Brain Plasticity and Alzheimer's Disease', 29 March 2013. Available at http://dementiatoday.com/brain-plasticity-and-alzheimers-disease-2/ (accessed 26 June 2017).

Erol, R., Brooker, D. and Peel, E. (2015) *Women and Dementia: A Global Research Review.* London Alzheimer's Disease International. Available at www.alz.co.uk/sites/default/files/pdfs/Women-and-Dementia. pdf (accessed 26 June 2017).

Fonda, J. (2012) *Prime Time: Love, Health, Sex, Fitness, Friendship, Spirit – Making the Most of All Your Life.* New York, NY: Random House.

Fruehwirth, R. (2016) *The Drawing of This Love: Growing in Faith with Julian of Norwich.* London: Canterbury Press Norwich.

Heyman, A. (2016) *Scary Old Sex.* New York, NY: Bloomsbury Publishing.

Hoogeveen, F.R. (2006) *The Last Taboo: Dementia, Intimacy and Sexuality.* Available at https://franshoogeveen.files.wordpress.com/2015/09/ intimacy_sexuality_frhoogeveen.pdf (accessed 18 July 2017).

Horstman, J. (2012) *The Scientific American Book of Love, Sex and the Brain. The Neuroscience of How, When, Why and Who We Love.* San Francisco, CA: John Wiley & Sons.

Howard, S (2014) *The Things Between Us. Living Words: Anthology 1 – Words and Poems of People Experiencing Dementia.* Edinburgh: Shoving Leopard.

Jong, E. (2015) *Fear of Dying.* New York, NY: St Martin's Press.

Juska, J. (2004) *A Round-Heeled Woman: My Late-Life Adventures in Sex and Romance.* New York, NY: Vintage.

Kitwood, T. (1997) *Dementia Reconsidered: The Person Comes First.* Buckingham: Open University Press.

Knocker, S. and Smith, A. (2017) *Safe to Be Me: Meeting the Needs of Older Lesbian, Gay, Bisexual and Transgender People Using Health and Social Care Services. A Resource Pack for Professionals.* London: Age UK in Partnership with Opening Doors London.

Knocker, S. (2012) *Perspectives on Ageing: Lesbians, Gay Men and Bisexuals.* York: Joseph Rowntree Foundation. Available at www.jrf.org. uk/report/perspectives-ageing-lesbians-gay-men-and-bisexuals (accessed 26 June 2017).

Koenig, H.G., George L.K. and Titus, P. (2004) 'Religion, spirituality and health in medically ill hospitalized older patients.' *Journal of the American Geriatrics Association 52,* 554–562.

Landinsky, D. (2002) *Love Poems from God: Twelve Sacred Voices from the East and West.* New York, NY: Penguin.

Leader, G., Litherland, R., Mason, T., Pitchick, T., Sansom, S. and Robertson, G. (2014). *Mindfulness and Dementia: Report of a Pilot Study.* A joint project by Innovations in Dementia and Positive Ageing Associates. Exeter: Innovations in Dementia CIC/Positive Ageing Associates.

Lee, D., Nazroo, J., O'Connor, D.B., Blake, M. and Pendleton, N. (2016) 'Sexual health and wellbeing among older men and women in England: Findings from the English Longitudinal Study of Ageing.' *Archives of Sexual Behavior 45,* 1, 133–144.

Lipinska, D. (2009) *Person-Centred Counselling for People with Dementia: Making Sense of Self.* London: Jessica Kingsley Publishers.

Long, D. (2014) 'Why Regular Sex May Actually Boost Brain Power.' *Huffpost,* 9 October 2014. Available at www.huffingtonpost. com/2014/10/09/sex-benefits-health-_n_5922574.html (accessed 26 June 2017).

Mackinlay, E. (ed.) (2010) *Ageing and Spirituality across Faiths and Cultures.* London: Jessica Kingsley Publishers.

Mackinlay, E. and Trevitt, C. (2012) *Finding Meaning in the Experience of Dementia: The Place of Spiritual Reminiscence Work.* London: Jessica Kingsley Publishers.

Mearns, D. and Thorne, B. (2000) *Person-Centred Therapy Today: New Frontiers in Theory and Practice.* London: Sage Publications.

Mitchell, G. (2016) *Doll Therapy in Dementia Care: Evidence and Practice.* London: Jessica Kingsley Publishers.

Power, G.A. (2014) *Dementia Beyond Disease: Enhancing Well-Being.* Baltimore, MD: Health Professional Press.

Rogers, C.R. (1951) *Client-Centred Therapy: Its Current Practice, Implications for Theory.* London: Constable.

Rogers, C.R. (1961) *On Becoming a Person.* Boston, MA: Houghton Mifflin.

Rogers, C.R. (1980) *A Way of Being.* Boston, MA: Houghton Mifflin.

Sawer, P. (2017) 'At the age of 90 and after death of beloved wife WWII veteran becomes a woman.' *The Telegraph.* Available online at www.telegraph.co.uk/news/2017/03/29/wwii-vet-becomes-woman-age-90-death-wife (accessed 19 July 2017).

Sheard, D. (2007) '"A Kiss is still a Kiss": People living with a dementia – Sexuality, Intimacy, Relationships and Closeness.' Module 11, An Emotional Journey: Person-Centred Culture Change Course. Brighton: Dementia Care Matters

Sparks, N. (1996) *The Notebook.* London: Doubleday.

Swaffer, K. (2016) *What the Hell Happened to My Brain?* London: Jessica Kingsley Publishers.

Tanner, L.J. (2017) *Embracing Touch in Dementia Care: A Person-Centred Approach to Touch and Relationships.* London: Jessica Kingsley Publishers.

Westwood, S. and Price, E. (eds) (2016) *Lesbian, Gay, Bisexual and Trans* Individuals Living with Dementia.* Abingdon: Routledge.

Whitman, L. (ed.) (2016) *People with Dementia Speak Out.* London: Jessica Kingsley Publishers.

Whitsed-Lipinska, D.M. (2001) 'Sexuality and older people.' *Signpost: Journal of Dementia and Mental Health Care of Older People 6,* 2, 11–12.

Whitsed-Lipinska, D.M. (2003) 'Sexually Speaking.' *Pathways: Newsletter of the Dementia Services Development Centre (DSDC),* article nos 8, 10, 12, 14. Stirling: Stirling University.

Further Resources

Acts and Policies

National Dementia Strategy 'Living Well with Dementia' (2009) Department of Health
www.gov.uk/government/publications/living-well-with-dementia-a-national-dementia-strategy

Mental Capacity Act (2005)
www.gov.uk/government/collections/mental-capacity-act-making-decisions

Deprivation of Liberty Safeguards (2009)
www.gov.uk/government/collections/dh-mental-capacity-act-2005-deprivation-of-liberty-safeguards

Human Rights Act (1998)
https://www.equalityhumanrights.com/en/human-rights/human-rights-act

Projects

'Over the Rainbow' Lesbians, Gay, Bisexual and Trans People and Dementia Project, February 2015. University of Worcester Association for Dementia Studies and DEEP.

Websites

Alzheimer's Association, Inside the Brain: An Interactive Tour
www.alz.org/alzheimers_disease_4719.asp

Sex and Intimate Relationships. Alzheimer's Society Fact Sheet
www.alzheimers.org.uk/download/downloads/id/1801/
factsheet_sex_and_intimate_relationships.pdf

Supporting lesbian, gay, bisexual people with dementia. Alzheimer's
Society Fact Sheet
www.alzheimers.org.uk/download/downloads/id/3555/
supporting_a_lesbian_gay_bisexual_or_trans_person_with_
dementia.pdf

The needs of older lesbians, gay men and transgender people
http://openingdoorslondon.org.uk

Pick's Disease
www.raredementiasupport.org

Rare Disease Support and Advice
www.raredisease.org.uk/supporters

Mind UK
www.mind.org.uk

BILD (British Institute of Learning Disabilities)
www.bild.org.uk

Care Quality Commission
www.cqc.org.uk